Florian Kowalke

The Tumour Suppressor Parafibromin and the Architecture of the hPaf1C

Florian Kowalke

The Tumour Suppressor Parafibromin and the Architecture of the hPaf1C

The role of a novel tumour suppressor in the development of cancer

Südwestdeutscher Verlag für Hochschulschriften

Impressum/Imprint (nur für Deutschland/ only for Germany)
Bibliografische Information der Deutschen Nationalbibliothek: Die Deutsche Nationalbibliothek verzeichnet diese Publikation in der Deutschen Nationalbibliografie; detaillierte bibliografische Daten sind im Internet über http://dnb.d-nb.de abrufbar.
Alle in diesem Buch genannten Marken und Produktnamen unterliegen warenzeichen-, markenoder patentrechtlichem Schutz bzw. sind Warenzeichen oder eingetragene Warenzeichen der jeweiligen Inhaber. Die Wiedergabe von Marken, Produktnamen, Gebrauchsnamen, Handelsnamen, Warenbezeichnungen u.s.w. in diesem Werk berechtigt auch ohne besondere Kennzeichnung nicht zu der Annahme, dass solche Namen im Sinne der Warenzeichen- und Markenschutzgesetzgebung als frei zu betrachten wären und daher von jedermann benutzt werden dürften.

Verlag: Südwestdeutscher Verlag für Hochschulschriften Aktiengesellschaft & Co. KG
Dudweiler Landstr. 99, 66123 Saarbrücken, Deutschland
Telefon +49 681 37 20 271-1, Telefax +49 681 37 20 271-0, Email: info@svh-verlag.de
Zugl.: Zürich, ETH Zürich, Dissertation, 2008

Herstellung in Deutschland:
Schaltungsdienst Lange o.H.G., Berlin
Books on Demand GmbH, Norderstedt
Reha GmbH, Saarbrücken
Amazon Distribution GmbH, Leipzig
ISBN: 978-3-8381-0682-3

Imprint (only for USA, GB)
Bibliographic information published by the Deutsche Nationalbibliothek: The Deutsche Nationalbibliothek lists this publication in the Deutsche Nationalbibliografie; detailed bibliographic data are available in the Internet at http://dnb.d-nb.de.
Any brand names and product names mentioned in this book are subject to trademark, brand or patent protection and are trademarks or registered trademarks of their respective holders. The use of brand names, product names, common names, trade names, product descriptions etc. even without a particular marking in this works is in no way to be construed to mean that such names may be regarded as unrestricted in respect of trademark and brand protection legislation and could thus be used by anyone.

Publisher:
Südwestdeutscher Verlag für Hochschulschriften Aktiengesellschaft & Co. KG
Dudweiler Landstr. 99, 66123 Saarbrücken, Germany
Phone +49 681 37 20 271-1, Fax +49 681 37 20 271-0, Email: info@svh-verlag.de

Copyright © 2009 by the author and Südwestdeutscher Verlag für Hochschulschriften Aktiengesellschaft & Co. KG and licensors
All rights reserved. Saarbrücken 2009

Printed in the U.S.A.
Printed in the U.K. by (see last page)
ISBN: 978-3-8381-0682-3

Für meine Eltern und Grosseltern,

die mir ein wundervolles Zuhause gaben,
die mich in Australien die englische Sprache erlernen liessen,
die mir die einzigartigen Erfahrungen in der Elfenbeinküste ermöglichten,
mir meinen ersten Computer schenkten,
mein Studium finanzierten.

Table of Contents

Table of Contents	II
Zusammenfassung:	1
Summary	3
Abbreviations	5
1 Introduction	12
1.1 Parathyroid Hyperplasia and Hyperparathyroidism Jaw Tumour syndrome (HPT-JT)	12
1.2 The yeast Paf1 complex (yPaf1C) and eukaryotic transcription	13
1.3 The components of the human Paf1C (hPaf1C)	17
1.4 Parafibromin	19
1.5 Aim of the project:	23
2 Results	24
2.1 The hPaf1C is a dense network of interactions between its five components	24
2.2 Generation of human cancer cell lines that inducibly and constitutively downregulate PFM	34
2.3 Knockout of Pfm in MEFs increases cell death and reduces the expression of genes involved in cell growth and proliferation	36
2.4 Generation of polyclonal antibodies against murine Pfm	43
3 Discussion	46
3.1 The Paf1 complex (hPaf1C) is a dense network of interactions between its five components	46
3.2 Generation of human cancer cell lines that inducibly and constitutively downregulate PFM	51
3.3 Knockout of Pfm in MEFs increases cell death and reduces the expression of genes involved in cell growth and proliferation	52
3.4 Generation of polyclonal antibodies against murine Pfm	54
4 Material and Methods	56
Part I: Material	56
4.1 General Chemicals and Material	56

4.2 Chemicals and Media used in Tissue Culture Experiments	58
4.3 Antibodies	59
4.4 Restriction Enzymes	60
4.5 Radiochemicals	60
4.6 Length standards (for proteins and DNA)	61
4.7 DNA Oligonucleotides	61
4.7.1 Oligonucleotides for Sequencing	61
4.7.2 Oligonucleotides for Cloning	62
4.7.3 Oligonucleotides for qRT-PCR	63
4.7.4 Oligonucleotides for antisense experiments	65
4.7.5 Oligonucleotides for genotyping	65
4.8 Plasmids	66
4.9 Bacterial strains	68
4.10 Mammalian Cell lines	68
4.11 Insect Cell lines	69
4.12 Viruses	69
Part II: Methods in Molecular Biology, Proteinbiochemistry, Cell Biology	71
4.13 Isolation of DNA	71
4.13.1 Isolation of plasmid DNA from bacterial cultures (Mini, Midi, Maxi)	71
4.13.2 Isolation of genomic DNA for genotyping of MEFs	72
4.13.3 Isolation of DNA from Agarose gels using the QIAEX II Agarose Gel Extraction Protocol	72
4.14 Isolation of RNA	73
4.15 Quantification of Nucleic Acids	73
4.16 Restriction enzyme digestions	74
4.17. Ligation of DNA fragments	74
4.17.1 Liquid Culture	74
4.17.2 Solid Culture	75
4.17.3 Transformation of bacteria	75
4.18 Preparation of competent Bacteria *E. coli* (DH5α)	75
4.19 Agarose Gel electrophoresis	76
4.20 Purification of proteins	76
4.20.1 Affinity purification using the GST-tag	76

4.20.2 Affinity purification using the MBP-tag 78
4.21 Purification of polyclonal antibodies against parafibromin 78
    4.21.1 Preparation of the affitnity column for antibody purification 78
    4.21.2 Purification and dialysis of polyclonal antibodies 79
4.22 DNA sequencing 79
4.23 PCR 79
    4.23.1 PCR 79
    4.23.2 Reverse transcriptase PCR 80
    4.23.3 Quantitative PCR 81
4.24 Cell Culture 81
    4.24.1 Cell culture of the immortalized insect cell *Sf9* 81
    4.24.2 Generation and amplification of Baculovirus 82
    4.24.3 Cell culture mammalian cell lines (splitting, freezing, thawing) 82
    4.24.4 Preparation of primary mouse embryonic fibroblasts 83
    4.24.5 Counting of mammalian and insect cells 84
    4.24.6 Retroviral transduction of mammalian cell lines and long-term storage of viruses 84
    4.24.7 Calcium-Phosphate Transfection of 293T cells to produce Lentivirus and infection of target cell lines 84
    4.24.8 Transfection of LinX cells to produce murine embyronic stem cell virus 85
    4.24.9 Generation of cell lines, which inducibly or stably downregulate Paf1C components 86
    4.24.10 Production of Adenovirus expressing Cre-recombinase 86
4.25 Isolation of proteins 87
4.26 Quantification of proteins 87
    4.26.1 Bradford Assay 87
    4.26.2 Colloidal Coomassie Staining 88
4.27 Production of polyclonal antibodies 88
4.28 Denaturing (SDS) discontinous Polyacrylamide gelelectrophoresis (PAGE) 88
4.29 Western Blotting and Immunodetection of proteins 89
    4.29.1 Odyssey system 89

4.30 Fluorescent Activated Cell Sorting (FACS)   89

4.31 *In vitro* Translation and pulldown of *in vitro* translates with GST fusion proteins   90

5 Acknowledgements   92

6 Bibliography   93

Zusammenfassung:

HRPT2 ist ein neues Tumorsuppressor-Gen welches in Nebenschilddrüsenkrebs, Nierenkrebs, Brustkrebs und Magenkrebs mutiert ist. HRPT2 besteht aus 17 Exonen und kodiert für das aus 531 Aminosäuren bestehendesProtein Parafibromin (PFM). Die Primärsequenz von PFM zeigt mässige Homologie (32% Identität) zu Cdc73, einem Protein aus der Bäckerhefe. Cdc73 ist Teil des Paf1 Komplexes (Paf1C), welcher verschiedene Schlüsselfunktionen in der Genexpression, vor allem während der Transkriptionselongation, übernimmt. Jüngere biochemische Studien konnten zeigen, dass PFM Teil des, zum Paf1C in der Bäckerhefe homologen, menschlichen Paf1C ist. Der menschliche Paf1C enthält neben PFM auch die Proteine Paf1, Ctr9, Leo1 und Ski8. Ausserdem ist bereits bekannt, dass PFM an das unkonventionelle Prefoldin URI, sowie die Histonmethylasekomplexe Set1 und Dot1, die Histonubiquitylierungsenzyme Bre1 und Rad6, unphosphorylierte sowie phosphorylierte Formen der RNA Polymerase II (RNAPII) sowie an β-Catenin durch Parafibromins β-Catenin-Interaktionsdomäne bindet.

Darüber hinaus konnte gezeigt werden, dass PFM einen negativen Einfluss auf den Zellzyklus hat, und dass PFM knockouts in Drosphila und Maus embryonisch lethal sind (vermutlich während des Schlüpfens der Blastozyste). Induzierte PFM knockouts führen *in vitro* zu Apoptose und *in vivo* innerhalb von drei Wochen zu verringerten Organgrössen und Kachexie (Auszehrung) (Wang, et al. 2008). Mittels Chromatin IP, identifizierten Wang et al. (2008) ferner die ersten direkten Zielgene von PFM in Mäuseembryofibroblastenzellen. Diese Zielgene sind H19, Igf1, Igf2, Igfbp4, Hmgcs2, Hmga1, and Hmga2. Zusammengefasst legen diese Ergebnisse die Vermutung nahe, dass PFM die Expression von solchen Genen bewirkt, deren Produkte Relevanz für Tumorunterdrückung und Apoptose besitzen.

In dieser Arbeit haben wir die molekulare Architektur des humanen Paf1C (hPaf1C) identifiziert. Anhand der Daten lässt sich zeigen, dass der hPaf1C eine hohe Dichte an direkten Protein-Protein Bindungen besitzt, und dass der N-terminale Teil von Paf1 sowie zu einem geringen Ausmass auch Ctr9, Ski8 und PFM das Zentrum dieses Proteinkomplexes bilden. Natürlich vorkommende, klinisch relevante

Punktmutationen von PFM haben keine nachweisbaren Auswirkungen auf die Protein-Protein Interaktionen zwischen PFM und den anderen Komponenten des hPaf1C. Im Gegensatz dazu zeigen wir in der vorliegenden Arbeit, dass die N-terminalen 222 Aminosäuren von PFM nicht in der Lage sind, ein Mitglied des hPaf1C zu binden. Da beinahe alle bekannten klinisch relevanten Mutationen in PFM die C-terminale Hälfte des Proteins betreffen, deuten unsere Erkenntnisse an, dass die Tumorsupressorfunktion von PFM abhängig vom hPaf1C ist. Interessanterweise konnten wir weiter zeigen, dass dieselbe PFM Domäne welche die Bindung zu β-Catenin vermittelt, auch für die Interaktion mit Paf1 und Ski8 notwendig ist. Ausserdem berichten wir zum ersten Mal, dass PFM zumindest *in vitro* in der Lage ist zu dimerisieren und dass PFM als einzige hPaf1C Komponente eine direkte Wechselwirkung mit URI eingehen kann.

Darüber hinaus haben wir zwei polyklonale Antikörper gegen murines Pfm hergestellt, sowie verschiedene Krebszelllinien, welche PFM konstitutiv oder induzierbar herunterregulieren. In keiner dieser Krebszelllinien konnten Phänotypen oder molekulare Veränderungen detektiert werden. Dagegen exprimieren im Rahmen dieser Arbeit hergestellte PFM[-/-] Mäuseembryofibroblasten nur noch deutlich verringerte Mengen der PFM Zielgene Igf1, Igf2, Hmg1 und Igfbp4, zeigen jedoch keine veränderte Aktivität im PI3K-Stoffwechselweg. Ferner können wir mit unseren Daten zeigen, dass eine Cre-abhängige Deletion von PFM in Mäuseembryofibroblasten zu Zelltod führt.

Summary

HRPT2 is a novel tumour suppressor gene that is lost in parathyroid cancer, renal cancers, breast cancer and gastric cancer. HRPT2 is comprised of 17 exons and encodes a predicted protein of 531 amino acids, termed parafibromin (PFM). The primary sequence of PFM displays modest homology (32% identity) to budding yeast Cdc73, a component of the Paf1 complex (Paf1C), which is thought to have key roles at various stages of the gene expression pathway, especially during transcriptional elongation. Recent biochemical studies in humans have demonstrated that PFM is present in the human protein complex homologue to yeast Paf1C. The hPaf1C comprises apart from PFM the proteins Paf1, Ctr9, Leo1 and Ski8. In addition, PFM has been shown to associate in complexes with the unconventional prefoldin URI, the histone methyltransferase complexes Set1 and Dot1, the histone ubiquitinating enzymes Bre1 and Rad6, with unphosphorylated as well as phosphorylated forms of RNA Polymerase II (RNAPII) GST-C-terminal domain (CTD) and with β-Catenin through its β-Catenin interaction domain.

Moreover, PFM has been reported to have a negative impact on cell cycle progression and that PFM knockouts in Drosphila and mouse are embryonic lethal (likely during hatching). Furthermore, induced knockout of PFM *in vitro* causes apoptosis and induced knockout of PFM *in vivo* reduces organ size and results in cachexia within 3 weeks *in vivo* (Wang et al. 2008). Using Chromatin IP, Wang et al. (2008) further reported the first known direct target genes of PFM in MEFs. These target genes are H19, Igf1, Igf2, Igfbp4, Hmgcs2, Hmga1, and Hmga2. Taken together, these findings strongly suggest that PFM contributes to the expression of genes whose products have relevancy in the suppression of tumour development and cell death.

In the present work, we identified the molecular architecture of the human Paf1C (hPaf1C). According to our data, the hPaf1C is rich in direct protein-protein interactions, and the N-terminal part of Paf1 as well as to a lesser extend Ctr9, Ski8 and PFM build the center of the human Paf1C (hPaf1C). Naturally occuring, clinically relevant point mutations of PFM do not disrupt any interaction between PFM and the other hPaf1C components. In contrast to that, we are able to show in the present work that the N-terminal 222 amino acids of PFM do not bind to any hPaf1C components. Since almost all known clinically relevant PFM mutations effect the expression of the C-terminal part of PFM, our findings provide evidence that the tumour supressor function of PFM is dependent on the hPaf1C. Interestingly, we further found that the same domain on PFM that is responsible for binding to β-Catenin mediates the interaction to Paf1 and Ski8 and report for the first time that PFM is able to dimerize *in vitro* and that it is the only hPaf1C component that directly interacts with URI.

Finally, we generated two polyclonal antibodies against murine Pfm as well as various cancer cell lines, which constitutively or inducibly downregulate PFM. None of those cell lines showed any phenotypes or molecular changes. $PFM^{-/-}$ MEFs generated during the course of this thesis however have a decreased expression of the PFM target genes Igf1, Igf2, Hmg1 and Igfbp4 but an unaltered activity of the PI3K-pathway. Last but not least, our data suggest that Cre-mediated deletion of PFM in MEFs causes in cell death.

Abbreviations

Abbreviation	Meaning
786-0	human renal cell carcinoma derived
°C	degrees Celcius
A	Ampère, absorption
aa	amino acid
AB	antibody
Amp	ampicilin
APS	Ammonium Persulfate
AY	Armelle Yart
Bcl-2	B-cell CLL/lymphoma 2
BRCA1/2	Breast cancer 1 or 2
bp	base pair
Blotto	TBST supplemented with 5% nonfat dried milk
BSA	Bovine Serum Albumin
C_T	Cycle Threshold
Cdc73	Cell division cycle 73 (yeast homologue of PFM)
Cdk7	Cyclin-dependent kinase 7
Cdk9	Cyclin-dependent kinase 9
cDNA	copy DNA
CID	β-Catenin Interaction Domain
cm	centimeter
COMPASS	COMplex of Protein ASsociated with Set1
conc.	concentration
CT	C-Terminus (of a protein) (whenever indicated, CT also stood for C-terminal part)
CTD	Carboxy terminal domain
CTDK-1	C-terminal Domain Kinase 1
CTK1	Catalytic (alpha) subunit of C-terminal domain kinase 1
Ctr9	Cyclin three-requiring protein 9

Ctrl	control
d	day(s)
D	Dilution factor
D. melanogaster	Drosophila melanogaster
Da	Dalton
DEPC	Diethylpyrocarbonate
dH$_2$O	destilled water (produced with Purelab Classic from ELGA)
DH5α	standard E. coli straion used in the lab
DMEM	Dulbecco's Modified Eagles Medium
DMP	Dimethyl Pimelimidate
DMSO	Dimethyl Sulfoxide
DNA	Desoxyribonucleic Acid
dNTP	desoxyribonucleotidetriphosphate
dox	Doxycycline
ds	double stranded
DTT	1,4-dithio-DL-threitol
E. coli	Escherichia coli
EDTA	Ethylenediaminetetraacetic Acid
e.g.	exempli gratia, for example
ES cells	Embryonic Stem cells
et al.	et alia, and others
etc.	etcetera
FACS	Fluorescent Activated Cell Sorting
FCS	Fetal Calf Serum
FK	Florian Kowalke
FL	Full Length
fl/fl	genotype indicating that the respective gene is flanked by two loxP sites
xg	X9.81m/s^2
g	gram
GAPDH	Glyceraldehyde-3-Phosphate Dehydrogenase
GSH	Glutathion

GSK3β	Glycogen Synthase Kinase 3β
GST	Glutathion-S-Transferase
h	hour
H. sapiens	*Homo sapies*
H2BK123MU	monoubiquitylated K123 of histone 2B
H3K4Me	methylation of histone 3 at K4
H3K36Me	methylation of histone 3 at K36
H3K79Me	methylation of histone 3 at K79
HDAC	histone deacetylase complex
HEK293	Human Embryonic Kidney derived cell line
HeLa	Henrietta Lacks (human cervix carcinoma derived cell line)
HIRA	Histone cell cycle regulation defective) homolog A
Hmga1	High mobility group AT-hook 1
Hmga2	High mobility group AT-hook 2
HMGCS2	3-Hydroxy-3-Methylglutaryl-Coenzyme A Synthase 2
HPA	Hepatopancreartic Ampulla
hPaf1C	human Paf1C
HPC1	Hereditary Prostate Cancer locus 1
HPT-JT	Hyperparathyroidism Jaw-Tumour Syndrome
HRPT2	Hyperparathyroidism 2 (gene encoding parafibromin)
hs	*homo sapiens*
ICS	"Institut Clinique de la Souris", Illkirch, France
IGF-I	Insulin-like Growth Factor 1
IGF-II	Insulin-like Growth Factor 2
IGFBP4	Insulin-like Growth Factor Binding Protein 4
IP	immunoprecipitation
IPTG	Isopropyl β-D-thiogalactopyranoside
incl.	including
IVT	*In vitro* Translation
k	kilo
K	one letter amino acid code for lysine
L	Liter

LB	Luria Bertani
LEF	Lymphoid Enhancer-binding Factor
LMP	MSCV/LTRmiR30-PIGΔRI
µ	Micro
m	mili or meter
M	molar (mol/L) or protein marker (in the figure legends)
MBP	Maltose Binding Protein
MEF	Mouse Embryonic Fibroblasts
min	minute
mm	*mus musculus*
mRNA	messenger RNA
MSCV	Murine Embryonic Stem Cell Virus
n	nano
NC	Nitrocellulose
NEB	New England Biolaboratories
NES	Nuclear Export Signal
NETN	NaCl, EDTA, Tris-Hcl, Nonidet P-40
NIH-3T3	National Institutes of Health 3-day Transfer, inoculum 3 x 10^5 cells; MEF derived cell line
NLS	Nuclear Localization Signal
NoLS	Nucleolar Localization Signal
NPC	Nuclear Pore Complex
NS	Non-Silencing
NT	N-Terminus (of a protein) (whenever indicated, NT also stood for C-terminal part)
OD	Optical Density
ON	Over Night
p150TSP	TPR-containing SH2-binding Phosphoprotein
P	one-letter amino acid code for proline
PAA	Polyacrylamide
Paf1	RNA-Polymerase II Associated Factor
Paf1C	Paf1 Complex
PAG	Polyacrylamide Gel

PAGE	Polyacrylamide Gel Electrophoresis
PBS	Phosphate-Buffered Saline
PBST	PBS supplemented with 0.2% Tween-20
PCR	Polymerase Chain Reaction
PD2	Pancreatic Differentiation 2
PDK1	Phosphoinositide Dependent Kinase 1
Pen/Strep	Penicillin/ Streptomycin
PFM	Parafibromin
PHDC	Pancreatic Head Ductal Carcinomas
pHPT	primary Hyperparathyroidism
PI	Propidium Iodide
PI3K	Phosphoinositide 3-Kinase
PMSF	Phenylmethylsulfonylfluorid
PRAD1	Parathyroid Adenomatosis 1; synonymous for Cyclin D1
PSBD	Paf1/ Ski8 Binding Domain
pSM2	plasmid Shag Magic 2
P-TEFb	Positive Transcription Elongation Factor b
QPCR	Quantitative PCR
qRT-PCR	quantitative RT-PCR
Ranbp2	Ran Binding Protein 2
RB	Retinoblastoma
RCC	clear cell Renal Cell Carcinoma
RE	Restriction Endonuclease
RMP	RBP5-Mediating Protein
Rn	*rattus norvegicus*
RNA	Ribonucleic Acid
RNAi	RNA interference
RNAPII	RNA Polymerase II
Rpb1	RNA polymerase II subunit 1
Rpb5	RNA polymerase II subunit 5
RPE-1	Retinal Primary Epithelia 1, human retinal epithelia derived
rpm	rounds per minute
RRL	Rabbit Reticulocyte Lysate

RT	Room Temperature
Rtf1	Restores TBP Function 1
RT-PCR	Reverse Transcriptase-PCR
rtTA	reverse transcriptional Transactivator
s	second
S	Swedberg/ one-letter amino acid code for serine
S.A.	Société Anonyme
S. cerevisiae	*Saccharomyces cerevisiae*
SDS	Sodium Dodecyl Sulfate
Ser	Serine
Sf9	*Spodoptera frugiperda* 9 (ovarian tissue derived)
SH2	Src-Homology 2
SH2BP1	SH2 domain Binding Protein 1
shRNA	small hairpin RNA
siRNA	small interfering RNA
Ski8	Superkiller protein 8
SkiC	Ski Complex
Spo11	Sporulation-specific protein 11
T	one-letter amino acid code for threonine
taq	*Thermus aquaticus* (thermostable)
TBE	Tris Borate EDTA
TBP	Tata box Binding Protein
TBST	Tris Buffered Saline Tween
TCF	T-Cell-specific transcription Factor
TEMED	(N,N,N',N'-Tetramethylethylene Diamine)
term.	Terminal
tet	Tetracycline
TFIIH	Transcription Factor (of RNAP) II H
Thr	Threonine
TMP	SIN-TREmiR30-PIGΔRI
TNN	Tween 20 NaOH Nonidet P40
TPR	TetratricoPeptide Repeat
tRNA	transfer RNA

TSG	Tumour Supressor Gene
U2OS	human bone osteosarcoma epithelia derived
URI	Unconventional prefoldin RPB5 Interactor
WB	western blotting/ western blot
WCE	Whole Cell Extract
Y	one-letter amino acid code for tyrosine
yPaf1C	yeast Paf1 Complex

1 Introduction

1.1 Parathyroid Hyperplasia and Hyperparathyroidism Jaw Tumour syndrome (HPT-JT)

HPT-JT is a rare (prevelance of 0.005% of all cancers (Hundahl, et al. 1999)) autosomal dominant disorder that was first described in 1990 (Cavaco, et al. 2004; Jackson, et al. 1990). The disease is characterized by primary hyperparathyroidism (pHPT, 80%), jaw tumours (mainly osteofibromas) (30-40%), polycystic kidney disease and other kidney tumours (incl.

Wilm's Tumour, mixed-epithelial-stromal tumour) (10%), parathyroid adenomas (50-75%) or carcinomas (15-40%), and less commonly with uterine tumours, pancreatic adenocarinomas, testicular mixed germ cell tumours, and Hurtle cell thyroid ademonas (Bradley, et al. 2005; Carling and Udelsman 2005; Cavaco, et al. 2001; Haven, et al. 2000; Jackson et al. 1990; Kakinuma, et al. 1994; Marx 2000; Marx, et al. 2002; Pimenta, et al. 2006; Simonds, et al. 2004; Tan and Teh 2004; Teh, et al. 1996; Wassif, et al. 1999). HPT-JT accounts for less than 1% of all pHPT, which may result from parathyroid adenomas, hyperplasia or carcinoma (Cavaco et al. 2001; Shane 2001). The usual treatment for parathyroid cancer is parathyroidectomy followed by careful monitoring of Ca^{2+} levels. It has a success rate of 95%.

Many familial cancers are caused by mutations in tumour suppressor genes (TSG), such as the BRCA1 and BRCA2 genes with 50%-80% lifetime risk for mutation carriers (Ford, et al. 1998). A hallmark for a classic TSG is loss of heterozygosity (LOH), or allelic imbalance in the tumour, where the wild-type allele is lost and the mutant retained. The hypothesis that it takes at least two mutations for a cancer to develop is often also referred to as Knudson's „two hit" hypothesis (Cavenee, et al. 1983; Knudson 1971; Nordling 1953). The precise molecular causes of parathyroid cancer is unknown, despite the fact that PRAD1/ Cyclin D1 is overexpressed in parathyroid adenomas and that it has been suggested to be an important driver for the development of parathyroid adenomas (Arnold, et al. 1989; Imanishi, et al. 2001). In additon, some studies have reported that loss of RB and loss as well as abnormalities of p53 play a role in the pathogenesis of parathyroid carcinomas (Cryns, et al. 1994a; Cryns, et al. 1994b; Subramaniam, et al. 1995).

Recently, the gene whose inactivation is directly associated with the pathogenesis of HPT-JT was identified as the *HRPT2* tumour suppressor gene, which contains of 17 exons and encodes a predicted protein of 531 amino acids, termed parafibromin (PFM) (Bradley et al. 2005; Carpten, et al. 2002; Tan, et al. 2004). The primary sequence of parafibromin displays 32% identity to budding yeast Cdc73, a component of the Paf1 complex, which is thought to have key roles at various stages of the gene expression pathway, especially during transcriptional elongation (Mueller and Jaehning 2002; Pokholok, et al. 2002; Rondon, et al. 2004; Squazzo, et al. 2002).

1.2 The yeast Paf1 complex (yPaf1C) and eukaryotic transcription

In yeast, the Paf1C is a highly abundant protein complex (15.000 – 30.000/ cell) and is directly associated to approximately 2% of all RNAPII molecules (Borggrefe, et al. 2001). The yPaf1C consists of its five members Paf1, Ctr9, Leo1, Cdc73 and Rtf1 (Betz, et al. 2002; Krogan, et al. 2002a; Mueller and Jaehning 2002; Pokholok et al. 2002; Porter, et al. 2002; Shi, et al. 1997; Shi, et al. 1996; Squazzo et al. 2002; Wade, et al. 1996). Ctr9 is with approximately 200.000 copies per cell one of the most abundant proteins in yeast (Mueller, et al. 2004). It has been described to be important for accurate chromosome segregation (Betz et al. 2002; Foreman and Davis 1996) and to be required for full expression of G1 type cyclins in *S. cerevisiae* (Betz et al. 2002; Koch, et al. 1999; Porter et al. 2002). In addition, Ctr9 knockouts have reduced levels of Leo1, Rtf1 and Cdc73 to 10%, and yeast strains lacking Paf1 also show reduced abundance of Rtf1 and Cdc73 levels (Mueller et al. 2004). A study by Chang et al. reported that *S. cerevisiae* strains deleted for Paf1 as well as those deleted for Cdc73 have increased recombination rates, reduced expression of genes involved in cell wall biosynthesis and are above that more sensitive to cell wall damages (Chang, et al. 1999). Furthermore, deletions of Paf1 and Cdc73 were reported to result in lower transcription efficiencies in yeast (Rondon et al. 2004), and Rtf1 and Cdc73 are required to link the other Paf1C components to chromatin (Mueller et al. 2004). Interestingly, Cdc73 has been shown to directly bind to the general transcriptional co-repressor TUP1, the yeast homologue of the histone chaperone factor HIRA (Kerkmann and Lehming 2001).

Transcription is a highly regulated process that is commonly separated into three phases, transcription initiation, elongation and termination. Each of those phases is firstly accompanied by specific phosphorylation patterns at the carboxy-terminal domain (CTD) of the largest RNAPII subunit (Rpb1) and secondly by covalent histone modifications. The Paf1C is considered to be a non-classical elongation factor, since deletion affects only a subset of genes in plants and yeast (Chang et al. 1999; He, et al. 2004; Mueller and Jaehning 2002; Oh, et al. 2004; Porter et al. 2002) and since it has been demonstrated to have roles in all three phases of transcription. During transcription initiation for instance, general transcription factors and RNAPII form the transcription initiation complex at the promoter. This complex contains an unphosphorylated CTD of RNAPII (**fig. 1.1a)**). The yPaf1C member yRtf1 is required for transcript start site selection (Stolinski, et al. 1997) and during the transition from transcription initiation to elongation. The kinases Kin28 as well as its human homologue Cdk7 belong to the respective TFIIH complexes and phosphorylate the heptapeptide repeats (YSPTSPS) of the CTD of RNAPII on Ser5 (Egloff and Murphy 2008; Gomes, et al. 2006; Komarnitsky, et al. 2000). This phosphorylation at Ser5 is an event that causes the dissociation of transcription initiation factors and the recruitment of transcription elongation factors including Set1 and the capping machinery (**fig. 1.1b)**) (Egloff and Murphy 2008; Komarnitsky et al. 2000; Schroeder, et al. 2000). The yPaf1C is also known to mediate the interaction between COMplex of Proteins ASsociated with Set1 (COMPASS) and RNAPII (Gerber and Shilatifard 2003; Ng, et al. 2003b). In yeast, yRtf1 and also yPaf1 are required for monoubiquitylation of histone 2B (H2BMU) at K123 (K120 on human H2B) (not shown), an event necessary for efficient transcription elongation as it removes the nucleosomal barrier (Chaudhary, et al. 2007). H2BMU is furthermore necessary for methylation of H3K4 (H3K4Me) by Set1 and of H3K79 (H3K79Me) by Dot1 (not shown) (Gerber and Shilatifard 2003; Laribee, et al. 2005; Ng, et al. 2003a; Wood, et al. 2003; Xiao, et al. 2005). Apart from yRtf1 and yPaf1, other components of the yPaf1C have been shown to be important for H3K4Me and K3K79Me. Accordingly, loss of yPaf1 and yCtr9 reduced H3K4Me levels and loss of yRtf1 and yPaf1 led to reduced H3K79Me levels (Krogan, et al. 2003a; Ng et al. 2003b).

During transcription elongation Ser5 phosphorylation of the CTD of RNAPII declines and the catalytic subunit of CDTK-1 (P-TEFb in mammals), CTK1 (Cdk9 in mammals) phosphorylates Ser2 of the CTD of RNAPII (**fig. 1.1c**)) (Cho, et al. 2001; Komarnitsky et al. 2000; Krogan, et al. 2002b; Krogan, et al. 2003b). This modification helps RNAPII to overcome initial elongation barriers and allows for termination and processing factors to associate with RNAPII (Egloff and Murphy 2008; Licatalosi, et al. 2002; Meinhart and Cramer 2004; Peterlin and Price 2006). The Paf1C plays a major role during the Ser2-phosphorylation of CTD as loss of yPaf1C components (Paf1 or Rtf1) lead to a reduction in RNAPII CTD Ser2 phosphorylation (Mueller et al. 2004; Nordick, et al. 2008; Penheiter, et al. 2005). During the course of transcription elongation, the Set1 complex translocates to the nascent RNA, freeing the Paf1C and thereby allowing it to recruit the Set2 complex (in a CTK1-dependent manner) (Hampsey and Reinberg 2003; Krogan et al. 2003b). The histone methylase complex Set2 then methylates Lys36 on histone H3 (H3K36Me) (**fig. 1.1d**) (Hampsey and Reinberg 2003; Krogan et al. 2003b), which is thought to lead to the recruitment of histone deacetylase complexes (HDACs), and thereby to the maintenance of a repressive chromatin structure (Carrozza, et al. 2005; Joshi and Struhl 2005; Keogh, et al. 2005). Above that, loss of yPaf1C results in shortened poly-A-tails and defective RNA 3'-end formation (Mueller et al. 2004; Nordick et al. 2008; Penheiter et al. 2005; Sheldon, et al. 2005). These defects have been suggested to be direct consequences of the changes in the pattern of CTD phosphorylation during transcription, as CTD phosphorylation defects are known to affect the ability of RNAPII to associate with factors regulating RNA synthesis, processing, packaging, and export (Bentley 2005; Jensen, et al. 2003; Proudfoot 2004; Sheldon et al. 2005).

Fig. 1.1

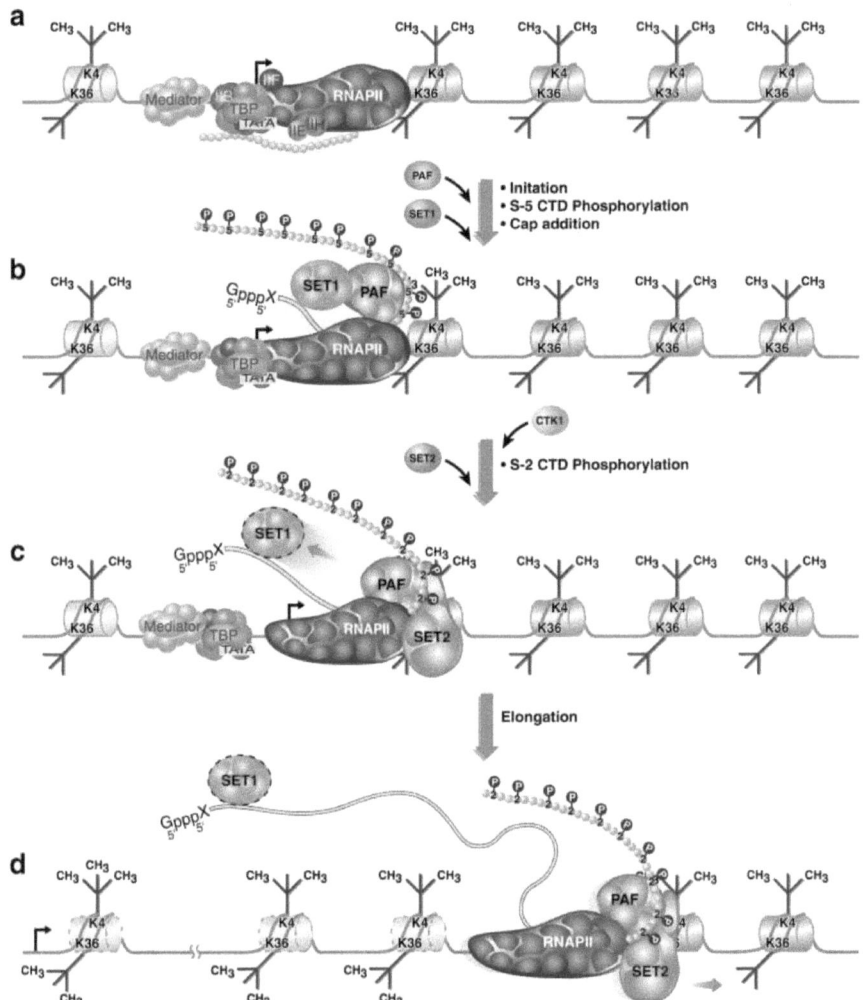

Fig. 1.1: A model of the interplay between CTD-phosphorylation and histone. The transcription cycle is a highly regulated process that is accompanied by an array of different modification patterns on histones and on the CTD of RNAPII. Many of those modifications are dependent on the Paf1C, which is believed to function as a central platform, coordinating the spacing and timing of many of the factors responsible for the modifications.
(adapted from Hampsey and Reinberg, 2003)

In summary, the yPaf1C is a recently discovered protein complex that regulates histone methylation and phosphorylation of RNAPII CTD, thereby coupling transcriptional with posttranscriptional events during mRNA synthesis.

1.3 The components of the human Paf1C (hPaf1C)

Homologues of all components of the yPaf1C exist in humans and all except for Rtf1 are also part of the hPaf1C (Rozenblatt-Rosen, et al. 2005; Yart, et al. 2005; Zhu, et al. 2005a; Zhu, et al. 2005b). Similarly to the yPaf1C, the human Paf1C (hPaf1C) associates with coding regions of genes and with transcriptionally active RNAPII (Rozenblatt-Rosen et al. 2005; Yart et al. 2005; Zhu et al. 2005a; Zhu et al. 2005b). The hPaf1C is above that also required to generate H2BMU, H3K4Me, and H3K79Me, demonstrating that at least parts of the function of yPaf1C are evolutionary conserved in humans (Rozenblatt-Rosen et al. 2005; Yart et al. 2005; Zhu et al. 2005a; Zhu et al. 2005b). Therefore, it has been suggested that similarly to the yPaf1C, the hPaf1C functions as a platform for co-transcriptional histone modifications and for factors involved in RNA biogenesis (surveillance, quality control, maturation and chromatin remodeling and modification) (Zhu et al. 2005b). Interestingly and despite the fact that *Drosophila* Rtf1 is not part of the *Drosophila* Paf1C, it associates with *Drosophila* Paf1 during transcription, facilitates Notch signalling, and interacts with SV40 large T antigen (Adelman, et al. 2006; Iwata, et al. 2007). Similarly, Rtf1 in zebrafish has been shown to facilitate Notch signalling (Akanuma, et al. 2007; Tenney, et al. 2006).

The hPaf1C does not contain Rtf1 but Ski8, which is also conserved across eukaryotes and is part of the Ski complex (SkiC) in *S. cerevisiae* as well as in *H. sapiens* (Zhu et al. 2005a). The Ski8C is a heterotrimeric complex that consists of Ski8, Ski2 and Ski3. In *S. cerevisiae*, the SkiC is required for 3'-5' mRNA decay and localizes to transcriptionally active genes in a Paf1C dependent manner (Zhu et al. 2005a). It has in addition to that been shown to protect the cell from viral replication by blocking synthesis of extrinsic mRNA transcripts (Widner and Wickner 1993). ySki8 also functions in meiotic recombination in complex with Spo11 in yeast – an observation that is especially interesting, as Paf1 and Cdc73 deleted yeast strains show increased recombination rates (Chang et al. 1999; Madrona and Wilson 2004). This function however seems not to be conserved in non-fungal eukaryotes (Jolivet, et al. 2006). hSki8 has been shown to be overexpressed in the pancreatic cell line Panc-1 (Chaudhary et al. 2007), and the chromosomal region to which the hSki8 gene localizes (15q25.1) is lost in colorectal cancer (Birkenkamp-Demtroder, et al. 2002) and in primary cutaneous B-cell lymphoma (Mao, et al. 2002).

A second component of the hPaf1C is the tetratricopeptide repeat protein Ctr9. The Ctr9 gene localizes to 11p15.3, a locus with chromosomal aberrations that have been linked to lung cancer and leukemia and is deleted in pancreatic cancer (Bashyam, et al. 2005; Redeker, et al. 1995). A knockout in zebrafish resulted in abnormal development of the heart, ears and neural crest cells (Akanuma et al. 2007).

hPaf1 was originally isolated as PD2, a gene overexpressed in human pancreatic adenocarcinoma, linking the third hPaf1C component (after Ski8 and Ctr9) to pancreatic hyperplasia (Chaudhary et al. 2007; Zhu et al. 2005a). As part of the amplicon 19q13, hPaf1 is known to be also overexpressed in Burkitt's Mantle cell and follicular lymphoma, lung cancer, breast cancer and uterine cancer (Curtis, et al. 1998; Moniaux, et al. 2006). It may be interesting to note that the putative oncogene AKT2 is present on the same amplicon and has been shown to be amplified and overexpressed in the following types of cancers: ovarian carcinomas (Bellacosa, et al. 1995; Cheng, et al. 1992), breast carcinomas (Bellacosa et al. 1995), pancreatic carcinomas (Cheng, et al. 1996; Miwa, et al. 1996; Ruggeri, et al. 1998), hepatocellular carcinoma (Xu, et al. 2004), and non-Hodgkin's lymphoma (Arranz, et al. 1996) (the amplification and overexpression of AKT2 is nicely reviewed in (Bellacosa, et al. 2005)).

A fourth component of the hPaf1C is hLeo1, a protein that is known to firstly bind to the E3 SUMO-protein ligase and nuclear pore complex (NPC) member Ranbp2 and secondly to β-Catenin (Mosimann, et al. 2006; Rozenblatt-Rosen et al. 2005). The gene locus of hLeo1 is amplified in colorectal cancer and malignant fibrous histiocytoma of the bone (Camps, et al. 2006; Tarkkanen, et al. 2006) and believed to harbour a potential osteosarcoma suppressor gene (Nathrath, et al. 2002).

In summary, the hPaf1C is a highly conserved eukaryotic protein complex that associates with transcribing RNAPII and functions as a platform for co-transcriptional histone modifications and a platform for RNAPII and its factors involved in RNA biogenesis. Moreover, the gene loci of every member of the hPaf1C are either amplified or lost in different types of hyperplasia. Due to those evidences and since only few functional links between hPaf1C components and hyperplasia have been established up to today, it is tempting to speculate that many roles of hPaf1C components in hyperplasia are structurally and functionally united by the hPaf1C.

1.4 Parafibromin

The fifth component of the hPaf1C and homologue of yeast Cdc73 is the recently discovered tumour suppressor parafibromin (Carpten et al. 2002; Howell, et al. 2003). Its mRNA (the unprocessed mRNA has a size of 2.7kbp) is encoded by the gene HRPT2, which has a size of 1.3 Mbp, consists of 17 exons and also encodes for an uncharacterized mRNA of 4.4kbp (Bradley et al. 2005; Carpten et al. 2002; Cavaco et al. 2004). The HRPT2 gene is part of the Hereditary Prostate Cancer Locus 1 (HPC1) (Sood, et al. 2001). This region has been linked to prostate cancer (Sood et al. 2001), and shown to be amplified in liver sarcoma (Parada, et al. 1998), non-brainstem glioblastoma (Korshunov, et al. 2005), breast cancer (Stange, et al. 2006), and in pancreatic head ductal carcinomas (PHDC) (Chang, et al. 2005). In contrast to that, the locus has been found to be lost in cancers of the hepatopancreatic ampulla (HPA) (Chang et al. 2005). Furthermore, parafibromin expression is lost in more than 60% of all cases of parathyroid cancer (Carpten et al. 2002; Howell et al. 2003; Tan et al. 2004), in renal cancers (12.5% of clear cell carcinomas, 21% of papillary carcinomas, 60% of chromophobe renal cell carcinomas, 38% of oncocytomas, 40% of Wilms tumours) (Zhao, et al. 2006), in breast cancer (more than 50%) (Selvarajan, et al. 2008), and in gastric cancer (Zheng, et al. 2008). In breast and gastric cancer, parafibromin expression was inversely correlated with tumour size, malignancy and survival (Selvarajan et al. 2008; Zheng et al. 2008).

Parafibromin shows a widespread expression in different tissues of mouse and human (e.g. in skin, kidney, heart, skeletal muscle, liver, testicals, parathyroid, spleen) but is not expressed in smooth muscle, connective tissue, hardly in pancreas (slightly in Langerhans cells), lymphnode, stomach, endothelium and some types of epithelia (thyroid, colon, uterine, tubaric, urinary, colonic) (Carpten et al. 2002; Porzionato, et al. 2006; Woodard, et al. 2004). PFM's localization to the nucleus and cytoplasm is tissue-dependent, confirming the different findings *in vitro* (Porzionato et al. 2006; Rozenblatt-Rosen et al. 2005; Yart et al. 2005; Zhang, et al. 2006).

The DNA sequence of parafibromin (PFM) is conserved and shows 32% identity and 47% homology to its yeast homologue Cdc73. The human form is identical to mouse and rat PFM and 58% identical to Hyrax, the PFM homologue in *D. melanogaster*. Several functional domains of PFM have been identified (**fig. 1.2**). Among those domains is a functional bipartite nuclear localization signal (NLS) between aa 126-139 (Bradley, et al. 2007; Hahn and Marsh 2005; Lin, et al. 2007; Rozenblatt-Rosen et al. 2005), three nucleolar localization signals (NoLS) between aa 76-92, 192-194, and 393-409 (Hahn and Marsh 2005), and three putative nuclear export signals (NES) (Hahn and Marsh, personal communication). Due to the slightly higher degree of conservation to Cdc73, the C-terminal part of parafibromin was named Cdc73 domain. The domain between aa 218 and 263 is called β-Catenin interaction domain (CID), as it was found to mediate the direct interaction to β-Catenin in *H. sapiens* and *D. melanogaster*. This interaction between PFM and β-Catenin seems interestingly to be required for nuclear transduction of the Wnt signal as RNAi against the *Drosophila* homologue of PFM, Hyrax, reduces transcriptional response of TCF/LEF binding sites (luciferase reporter) and of Wnt target genes (Mosimann et al. 2006). Surprisingly, the Wnt target gene c-myc has been reported to be upregulated upon RNAi-mediated inhibition of PFM or Paf1 expression in different human cancer cell lines (Lin, et al. 2008). Up to now, several dozen different mutations in HRPT2 have been described in various forms of hyperplasia. Almost all of those are frameshift mutations yielding truncated versions of PFM that hardly ever extend to aa 222 (Carpten et al. 2002; Cavaco et al. 2004; Cetani, et al. 2004; Haven, et al. 2007; Howell et al. 2003; Pimenta et al. 2006; Shattuck, et al. 2003; Simonds et al. 2004; Villablanca, et al. 2004; Warner, et al. 2004; Yart et al. 2005; Zhao et al. 2006). In addition to that, the following six different point mutations have been reported: M1L, K34Q, L64P, L253V, R292K, D379N (Carpten et al. 2002; Zhao et al. 2006). The most N-terminal PFM point mutation, PFM M1L, is a point mutation in the start codon that prevents translation of the whole protein (Carpten et al. 2002). PFM K34Q has been found in a clear cell renal cell carcinoma (RCC) and was, similarly to PFM L64P, shown to be defective in Cyclin D1 suppression (Woodard et al. 2004; Zhao et al. 2006). It can be speculated that PFM L64P exibits its effect due to the significant structural changes involved in replacing a leucine for a proline. The last three point mutations (L253V, R292K, D379N) are all located between aa 226 and 413, a part which has been shown to be involved in binding to other components of the hPaf1C (Rozenblatt-Rosen et al. 2005; Yart et al. 2005). It is furthermore worth to note that PFM L253V lies within the CID. The fifth point mutation of PFM, PFM R292K, has been discovered in Wilms tumour and is part of a yet unknown highly conserved domain (**fig. 1.2**) (Zhao et al. 2006). The most C-terminal mutation, PFM D379N, is positioned at the beginning of the conserved Cdc73 domain of PFM. **Fig. 1.2** gives an overview of the functional domains and point mutations of parafibromin.

Moreover, PFM has been shown to interact with several other interesting proteins. Among those is the direct interaction with the SV40 large T antigen (Iwata et al. 2007) and the interaction with the unconventional prefoldin URI (Gstaiger, et al. 2003; Yart et al. 2005), the histone methyltransferase complexes Set1 and Dot1, the histone ubiquitinating enzymes Bre1 and Rad6, and the unphosphorylated as well as phosphorylated forms of RNA Polymerase II (RNAPII) (Rozenblatt-Rosen et al. 2005; Yart et al. 2005).

RNAi-mediated downregulation of PFM in HeLa cells promotes S-Phase entry (Lin et al. 2008; Yart et al. 2005) and overexpression of parafibromin in HEK293 cells or MEFs results in the inhibition of proliferation (Iwata et al. 2007; Zhang et al. 2006). These findings are in line with a role of PFM as a potential tumour suppressor function. In cells expressing SV40 large T antigen however, it was surprisingly reported that PFM enhances cell growth (Iwata et al. 2007).

Fig. 1.2

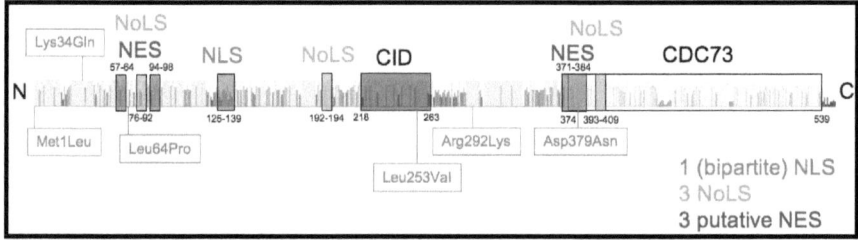

Fig. 1.2: **Alignment and functional domains of parafibromin.** Each yellow line represents an amino acid (aa) of parafibromin. The longer the line and the more yellow, the more conserved is the respective amino acid among the different species. PFM contains a bipartite NLS, three putative NES and three NoLS. In addition to that, a β-catenin interaction domain (CID) and a Cdc73 domain has been described. The locations of the six clinically relevant PFM point mutations that are currently known are also shown in the figure. The six species used for the homology search were: *Homo sapiens, Mus musculus, Rattus norvegicus, Bos taurus, Drosophila melanogaster, Caenorhabditis elegans*, and *Xenopus laevi*.
N: N-terminus
C: C-terminus

Conflicting reports have been published on the role of PFM in apoptosis. While Lin et. al (2007) reported that overexpression of PFM in NIH-3T3 cells induces while downregulation of PFM prevents apoptosis, another study suggested that knockout of parafibromin in primary MEFs (by Cre-recombinase) results in apoptosis (Wang et al. 2008). PFM knockouts in *D. melanogaster* and *M. musculus* have been reported to be embryonic lethal (likely during hatching) (Mosimann et al. 2006; Wang et al. 2008). Above that, induced downregulation of PFM in mice reduces sizes of organs and results in cachexia within three weeks, showing that PFM is an essential protein (Wang et al. 2008). Using Chromatin IP in MEFs, Wang et al. (2008) furthermore reported the discovery of the first direct target genes of PFM. These target genes are H19, Igf1, Igf2, Igfbp4, Hmgcs2, Hmga1, and Hmga2 (Wang et al. 2008). Since IGFs are required for normal prenatal and postnatal growth, reduced IGF expression upon PFM knockout could explain some of the phenotypes observed (Kooijman 2006).

1.5 Aim of the project:

Taken together, these findings suggest that PFM contributes to the expression of genes whose products have relevancy in tumour development and apoptosis. It is conceivable that part of its tumour suppressor function is mediated by the interactions of PFM with RNAPII, human Paf1C components and chromatin remodeling enzymes. Despite the fact that the first direct target genes of PFM have been discovered, the molecular mechanisms by which parafibromin acts upon them remains unclear. The aim of the present work was to identify the molecular architecture of the hPaf1C. We focussed on the regions of hPaf1C components, which are especially important for the integrity of hPaf1C. Apart from that, we wanted to analyze, if any of the known PFM point mutations disrupts binding to members of the hPaf1C and if the PFM domains responsible for binding to members of the hPaf1C overlap with parts of PFM that harbour its tumour supressor function. In addition to that, we wanted to generate various cell lines that constitutively and inducibly downregulate PFM in order to identify further functions of PFM by analyzing the effects of PFM loss-of-function at the cellular level.

2 Results

2.1 The hPaf1C is a dense network of interactions between its five components

In the first project, we studied the molecular architecture of the hPaf1C where we identified a dense network of direct interactions between its five core components. In our model, the N-terminal part of Paf1 forms the center of the hPaf1C, as it associates with all of the other hPaf1C components tested. Point mutants of PFM showed no altered binding abilities. In addition, we found *in vitro* evidence for the formation of PFM homo dimers and could show that PFM directly interacts with URI.

Identification of direct protein-protein interactions and the domains responsible for such bindings, can best be studied using immobilized GST fusion proteins to pull down *in vitro* translates of potential binding partners. To this end, cDNAs of hPaf1C components were cloned into the baculovirus transfer vector pAcGHLT-A before they were integrated into baculovirus genome to produce high amounts of GST fusion proteins in baculovirus infected *Sf9* cells. Glutathione beads were used to specifically pull down the five GST-tagged hPaf1C components before they were separated on a polyacrylamide gel (PAG) and detected by western blotting (WB) and immunostaining or by Coomassie staining (**fig. 2.1**). Using this procedure, all hPaf1C components were expressed as GST fusion proteins and purified in high amounts.

Fig. 2.1a) b)

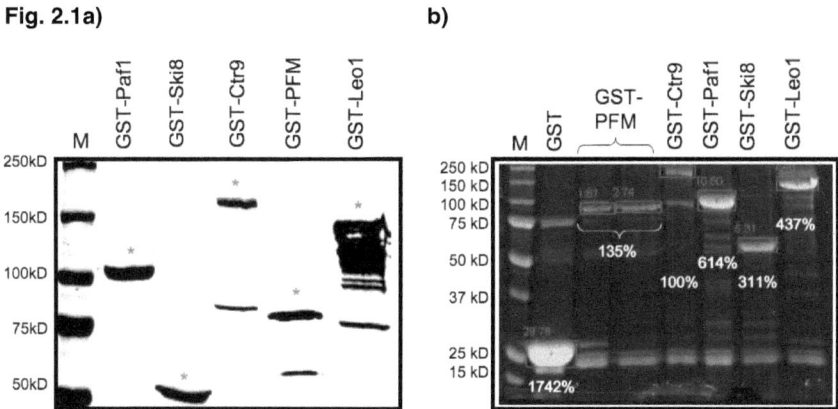

Fig. 2.1: GST and GST tagged versions of all hPaf1C components can be expressed in *Sf9* cells and purified with GSH beads. *Sf9* cells were infected with baculovirus harbouring an expression cassette for GST fusion proteins of hPaf1C components. The expressed GST fusion proteins as well as GST alone were purified using GSH-coupled beads and separated by polyacrylamide gel electrophoresis (PAGE). **a)** WB and immuno staining with a primary antibody against GST and **b)** coomassie staining of the polyacrylamide gels showed that all components were expressed in high amounts. Coomassie staining was used to equilibrate the amounts of protein for the subsequent *in vitro* binding assays.
M: protein marker

In order to identify direct binding partners within the hPaf1C, the amounts of GST fusion proteins were equilibrated and each GST fusion protein was then tested for its ability to pull down each of the five *in vitro* translated and ^{35}S radio-labelled hPaf1C components. The results are shown in **fig. 2.2** and place hPaf1 in the center of the complex, as *in vitro* translated Paf1 directly bound to all of other GST-hPaf1C components (**fig. 2.2a)**). *In vitro* translated PFM bound to GST-Ctr9, GST-Paf1 and to GST-Ski8 (**fig. 2.2b)**), while *in vitro* translated Ski8 could only be pulled down by GST-Ctr9 (**fig. 2.2c)**). *In vitro* translated Leo1 only bound to GST-Paf1 beads (**fig. 2.2d)**), while *in vitro* translated Ctr9 bound to all GST tagged fusion proteins except for GST-Leo1 (**fig. 2.2e)**).

Fig. 2.2a)

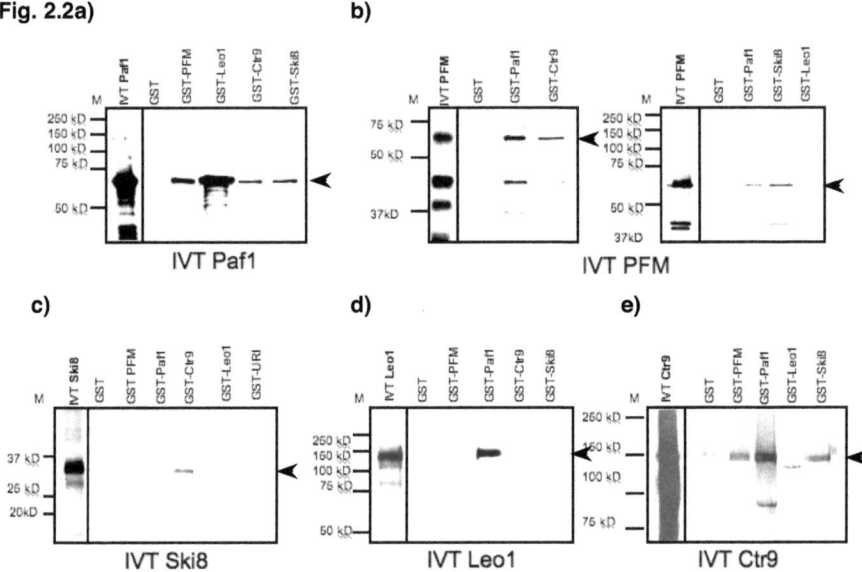

Fig. 2.2: The human Paf1 complex (hPaf1C) is a dense network of interactions between its five core components. GST tagged fusion proteins of the five hPaf1C components were produced in baculovirus-infected *Sf9* cells and used as baits on sepharose beads to pull down any other *in vitro* translated, radioactively labeled hPaf1C component. **a)** *In vitro* translated Paf1 could be pulled down by all other GST-hPaf1C components, but not by GST alone. **b)** *In vitro* translated PFM was pulled down by GST-Paf1, GST-Ctr9, and GST-Ski8 but neither by GST nor by GST-Leo1. **c)** *In vitro* translated Ski8 specifically bound to GST-Ctr9, but not to any other hPaf1C component or to GST alone. **d)** *In vitro* translated Leo1 directly bound to immobilized GST-Paf1, but not to any other hPaf1C component or GST alone. **e)** With the exception of GST-Leo1, *in vitro* translated Ctr9 was pulled down by all GST-hPaf1C components, demonstrating direct binding of Ctr9 to GST-PFM, GST-Paf1 and GST-Ski8 but not to GST alone. Arrow points indicate the expected sizes of *in vitro* translated proteins.

In the course of these binding studies we also found that PFM can bind to itself (**fig. 2.3**).

Fig. 2.3

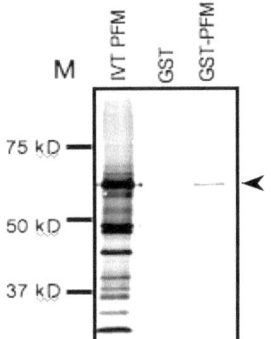

Fig. 2.3: PFM binds to itself *in vitro*. GST tagged PFM was produced in baculovirus-infected *Sf9* cells and used as a bait on sepharose beads to pull down, radioactively labeled *in vitro* translated PFM. GST-PFM was able to bind to *in vitro* translated PFM demonstrating the ability of PFM to dimerize.
M: protein marker

Furthermore, we knew from previous studies that PFM co-immunoprecipitates with URI (Rozenblatt-Rosen et al. 2005; Yart et al. 2005). We used the *in vitro* binding assay to test for direct interactions between URI and any hPaf1C component. From all five GST-hPaf1C components expressed (GST-Paf1, GST-Ctr9, GST-PFM, GST-Ski8 and GST-Leo1), an interaction was observed only between GST-PFM and URI (**fig. 2.4a**). This interaction was independent of whether PFM or URI was used as bait (**fig. 2.4**).

Fig. 2.4a)   b)

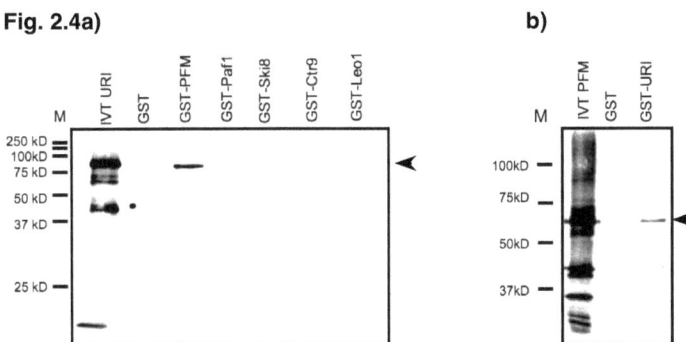

Fig. 2.4: URI directly binds to PFM but not to any other hPaf1C component *in vitro*. GST tagged fusion proteins of the five hPaf1C components were produced in baculovirus-infected *Sf9* cells and used as baits on sepharose beads to pull down *in vitro* translated, radioactively labeled URI. **a)** *In vitro* translated URI could be pulled down by *Sf9* cell expressed GST-PFM, but not by any other hPaf1C component. **b)** This interaction between PFM and URI was also confirmed with in vitro translated PFM that was pulled down by GST-URI.
M: protein marker

On the basis of our findings, we have integrated all direct interactions within the hPaf1C into a model, which is shown in **Fig. 2.5**. Each arrow in the model points from the *in vitro* translated protein to the GST tagged *Sf9* cell expressed protein. For instance, Leo1 directly interacts with Paf1 wether Leo1 is *in vitro* translated and pulled down by GST-Paf1 or *vice versa*.

Fig. 2.5

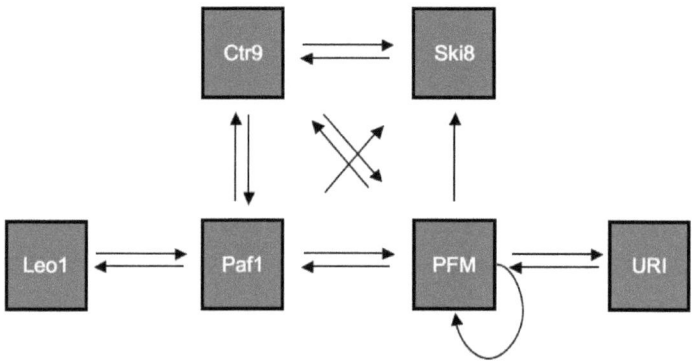

Fig. 2.5: The direct protein interaction map of the hPaf1C and URI. Our *in vitro* studies demonstrate a high number of direct interactions among the hPaf1C components. With the exception of Leo1, each hPaf1C component directly interacts with one another. URI is associated to the Paf1C via parafibromin and PFM and PFM is able to form homomers.

In subsequent steps, we analyzed the known clinically relevant point mutations of PFM (K34Q, L64P, R292K, D379N) for their ability to retain the interactions with GST-PFM, other GST-hPaf1C components and with GST-URI. We found that none of the point mutations had an altered binding ability to any protein tested (**fig. 2.6**).

Fig 2.6

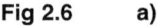

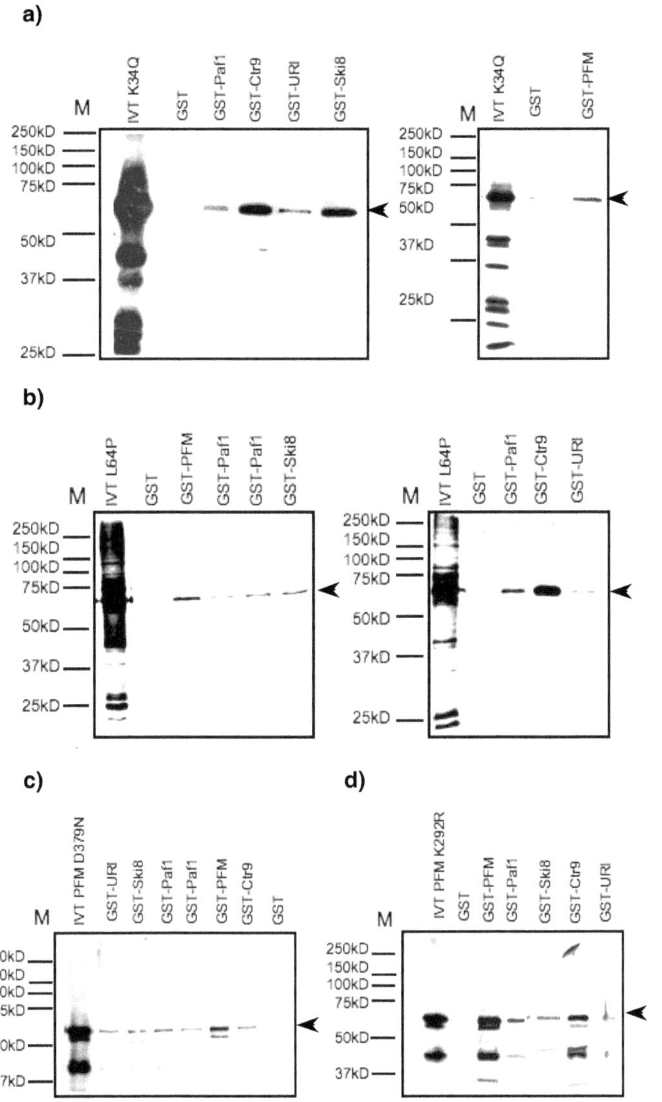

Fig. 2.6: **PFM point mutants can still bind to GST-PFM, GST-URI, GST-Ski8, GST-Paf1, and GST-Ctr9.** GST tagged fusion proteins of the five hPaf1C components and URI were produced in baculovirus-infected *Sf9* cells and used as baits on sepharose beads to pull down the four *in vitro* translated, radioactively labeled PFM point mutations. *In vitro*-translated **a)** PFM K34Q, **b)** PFM L64P, **c)** PFM D379N, **d)** PFM K292R were bound by GST-PFM, GST-URI, GST-Ski8, GST-Paf1, and GST-Ctr9 but not by GST.
M: protein marker

Most of the currently known clincially relevant mutations lead to N-terminally truncated versions of PFM that are shorter than 222 aa (Wang, et al. 2005) (i.e. shorter than PFM R222X), suggesting that the main tumour suppressor functions of PFM are located at a more C-terminal part (aa 222-531) of the protein. At the same time, the functions of the first 222 aa of PFM still remain to be discovered. In an attempt to understand if the abilities of N-terminally truncated PFM versions to bind members of the hPaf1C are effected by the truncations, we used PFM R222X in our binding assay (baits from the same preparations as in **fig. 2.2** were used). As shown in **Fig. 2.7**, PFM R222X neither binds to URI, nor to any hPaf1C component *in vitro*.

Fig. 2.7

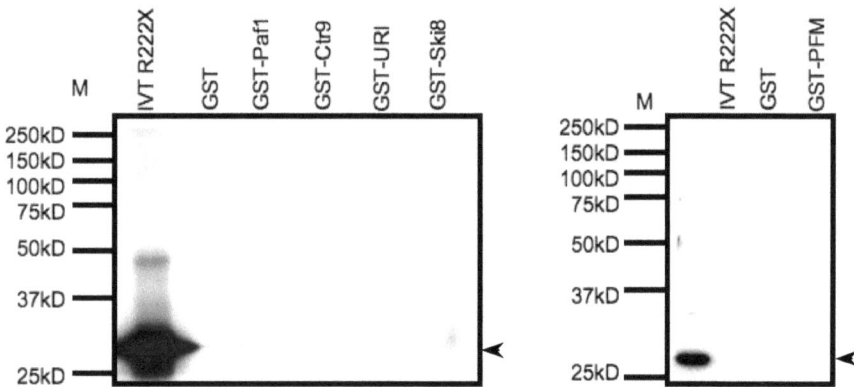

Fig. 2.7: The N-terminal 222 aa of PFM (PFM R222X) cannot be pulled down by hPaf1C component or by URI. GST tagged fusion proteins of the five hPaf1C components and URI were produced in baculovirus-infected *Sf9* cells and used as baits on sepharose beads to pull down *in vitro* translated, radioactively labeled PFM R222X. *In vitro*-translated PFM R222X, does not bind to Sf9 cell expressed GST-Paf1, GST-Ctr9, GST-URI, GST-Ski8 and GST-PFM.
M: protein marker

To further characterize the molecular architecture of the hPaf1C, the C- and N-terminal halfs of hPaf1, hCtr9 and PFM were cloned in front of a T7 promoter. Then, the N-terminal part, C-terminal part and FL of the three hPaf1C components were radioactively labelled using *in vitro* translation and tested for the ability to bind to any of the *Sf9* cell expressed GST-hPaf1C components. In the first set of experiments *in vitro* translated Paf1 and its halves were tested for their ability to bind to GST-Leo1,

GST-Ctr9 and GST-Ski8. As seen in **Fig. 2.8**, GST-Leo1, GST-Ctr9, and GST-Ski8 all bound as expected to the FL of Paf1 as well as to the N-terminal part of Paf1 but not its C-terminal part.

Fig. 2.8a) b) c)

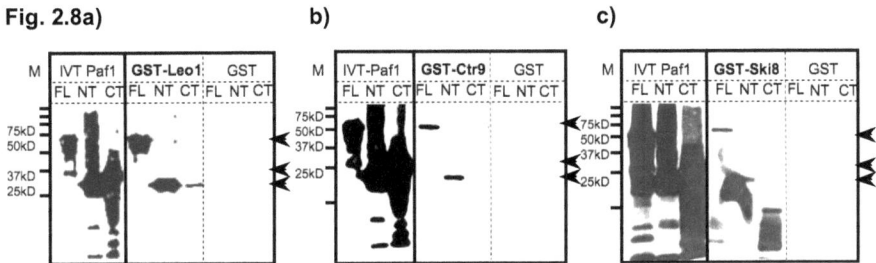

Fig. 2.8: **The N-terminal part of Paf1 binds to GST-Leo1, GST-Ctr9 and GST-Ski8.** GST tagged Leo1, Ctr9, and Ski8 were produced in baculovirus-infected *Sf9* cells and used as baits on sepharose beads to pull down the *in vitro* translated, radioactively labeled Paf1 FL, NT, and CT. *In vitro* translated N-terminal Paf1 but not C-terminal Paf1 was pulled down by **a)** GST-Leo1, **b)** GST-Ctr9 and **c)** GST-Ski8.
M: protein marker
FL: full length
NT: N-terminal part
CT: C-terminal part

In a second set of experiments, we *in vitro* translated Ctr9-FL, -NT, and -C-terminal part and tested for their abilities to be pulled down by GST-Paf1, GST-Ski8, and GST-PFM. The *in vitro* translated NT but not the C-terminal part of Ctr9 could be pulled down by Paf1 and Ski8. In contrast to that, GST-PFM pulled down both *in vitro* translated halves of Ctr9, indicating that there are at least two points of direct interaction between PFM and Ctr9 (**fig. 2.9**).

Thirdly, we tested PFM-FL, -N-terminal part, and -C-terminal part in our binding assay with GST-Paf and GST-Ski8. *In vitro* translated FL-PFM and the N-terminal part but not the C-terminal part of PFM bind to *Sf9* cell expressed GST-Paf1 and GST-Ski8 (**fig. 2.10**).

Fig. 2.9a)   **b)**   **c)**

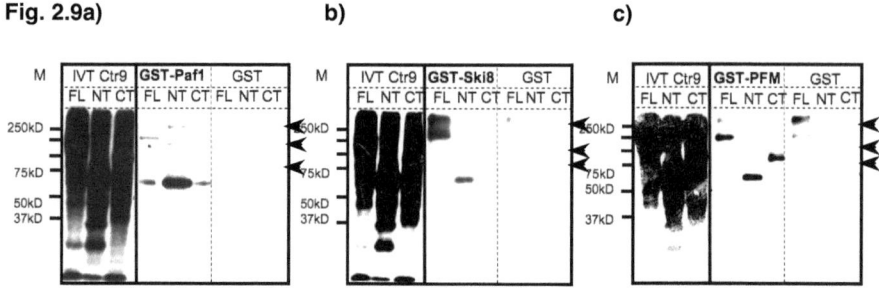

Fig. 2.9: The N-terminal part of Ctr9 binds to GST-Paf1, GST-Ski8 and GST-PFM. GST tagged Paf1, Ski8, and PFM were produced in baculovirus-infected *Sf9* cells and used as baits on sepharose beads to pull down the *in vitro* translated, radioactively labeled Ctr9 FL, NT, and CT. *In vitro* translated N-terminal Ctr9 but not C-terminal Paf1 was pulled down by **a)** GST-Paf1, and **b)** GST-Ski8. **c)** The NT as well as the CT of Ctr9 was reproducibly pulled down by GST-PFM.
M: protein marker
FL: full length
NT: N-terminal part
CT: C-terminal part

Fig. 2.10a)   **b)**

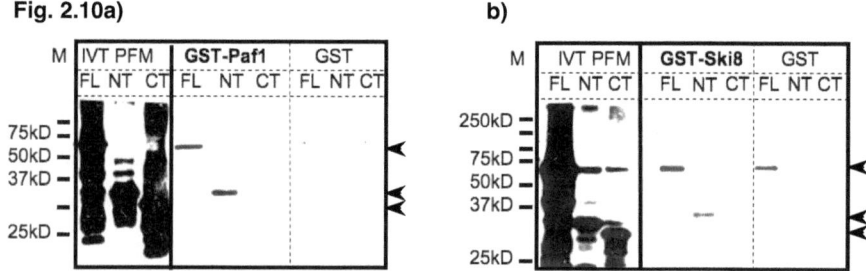

Fig. 2.10: The N-terminal part of PFM binds to GST-Paf1 and GST-Ski8. GST tagged Paf1 and Ski8 were produced in baculovirus-infected *Sf9* cells and used as baits on sepharose beads to pull down the *in vitro* translated, radioactively labeled PFM FL, NT, and CT. *In vitro* translated N-terminal but not C-terminal PFM was pulled down by **a)** GST-Paf1 and **b)** GST-Ski8.
M: protein marker
FL: full length
NT: N-terminal part
CT: C-terminal part

To our knowledge, this is the first systematic report on the interactions within the haf1C. Based on our results, we have developed a model of the molecular architecture of the hPaf1C (**fig. 2.11**). In that model, the N-terminal part of Paf1 and to a lesser extend also Ctr9, Ski8 and PFM build a robustly interlinked center of the complex that directly interacts with Leo1. Since none of the hPaf1C components interact with PFM R222X, but since GST-Ski8 and GST-Paf1 are able to pull down the *in vitro* translated N-terminal part of PFM (aa 1-270), we conclude that the domain between aa 222 and 270 of PFM mediates the interaction to Ski8 and to Paf1.

Fig. 2.11

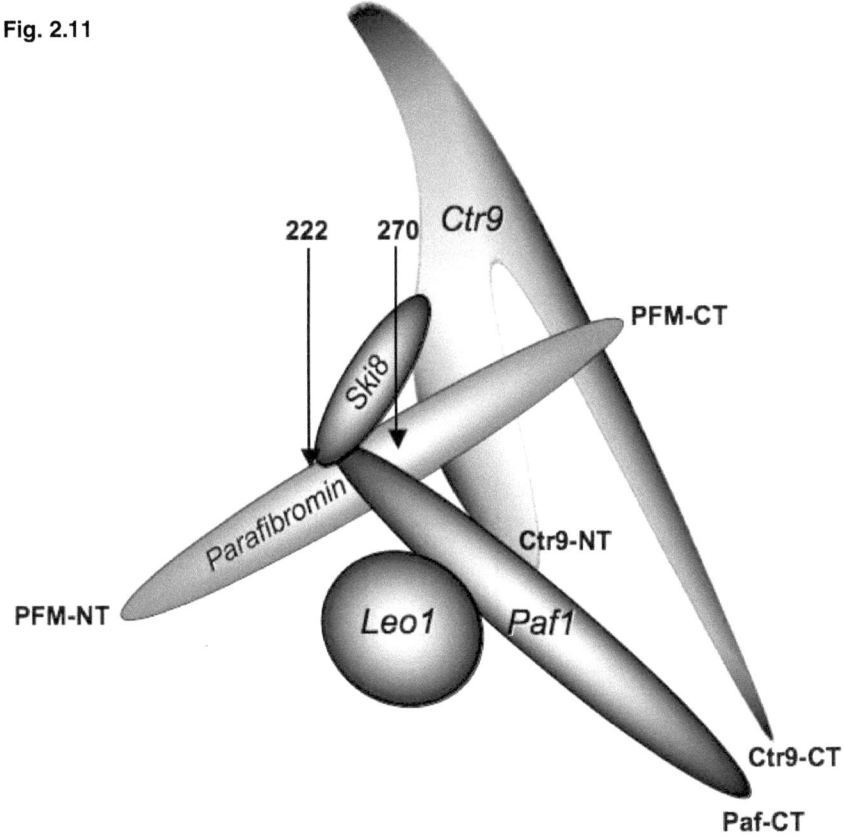

Fig. 2.11: The molecular architecture of the hPaf1 Complex. The Paf1C is built up of a dense network of interactions between it's five components Leo1, Paf1, Ski8, Ctr9 and PFM. In that model, the N-terminal part of Paf1 can be placed in the center of the complex as it interacts with Leo1, Ctr9, and Ski8. The N-terminal part of PFM interacts with Ski8, Paf1, and the N- and CT of Ctr9, and the N-terminal part of Ctr9 binds to Paf1, Ski8 and PFM.
CT: C-terminal part
NT: N-terminal part

2.2 Generation of human cancer cell lines that inducibly and constitutively downregulate PFM

In order to identify cell biological functions of PFM, we used retrovirus-mediated transfection of shRNA expression cassettes directed against all hPaf1C components to generate different human cancer cell lines that downregulate PFM, Ski8, Ctr9, and Leo1 on mRNA and protein levels.

In a first step, we generated cell lines, which constitutively downregulate PFM, Ctr9, Ski8 or Leo1. As shown by quantitative western blot and QPCR, expression of the respective target was reduced to 10-30% of original protein and mRNA levels in infected HeLa cell lines (**fig. 2.12**).

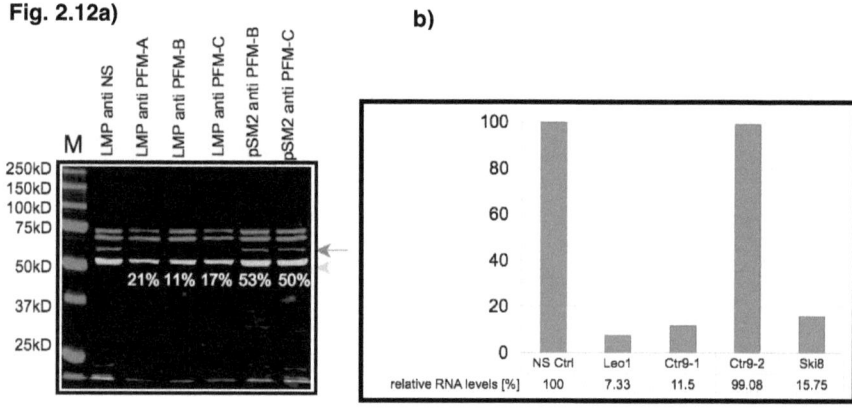

Fig. 2.12: Quantitative western blot and QPCR of mRNA of HeLa cell lines, which constitutively downregulate hPaf1C components. A retrovirus-mediated transfection of shRNA expression cassettes directed against hPaf1C components was used to generate HeLa cell lines, which constitutively downregulate PFM, Ctr9, Ski8 or Leo1. **a)** Western blot of cell lines constitutively downregulating PFM by three different hairpins (PFM-A, -B and -C) in two different retrovirus backbones (pSM2 and LMP). Cells infected with viral constructs harbouring one of three hairpins against PFM (PFM-A, -B, and -C) showed a decreased intensity of the PFM band (red, indicated by red arrow) compared to cells that had been infected with viral constructs harbouring the non-silencing hairpin (anti NS). The intensity of the tubulin band remained unchanged (green, indicated by the green arrow). Constructs of the pSM2 kind were less efficient in downregulating the PFM band (lanes 6 and 7). **b)** Quantitative measurement of RNA content in different HeLa cell lines constitutively downregulating Leo1, Ctr9, Ski8 and PFM in the LMP retrovirus backbone. Primers against 18S rRNA were used to normalize RNA amounts. Two different hairpins were used to downregulate Ctr9. In contrast to hairpin "Ctr9-1", hairpin "Ctr9-2" did not effectively downregulate Ctr9.
M: protein marker

With a similar approach we obtained kidney (786-0) and retinal (RPE-1) cell lines that constitutively downregulate PFM (data not shown). None of those cell lines showed any obvious phenotype. In order to see if the lack of a clear phenotype of cells downregulating PFM was dependent on the culturing time, we decided to generate cell lines that inducibly downregulate PFM. To this end, we cloned the same haripins into retroviral vectors containing a tetracycline response element and used the Tet-On-system in U2OS-cells. U2OS cells, which constitutively express the reverse tetracycline responsive transactivator (rtTA), were then infected with retrovirus (murine embryonic stem cell virus) that harboured functional shRNA against PFM under control of a tetracycline response element. After infection, cells were selected with puromycin (to select for cells containing the shRNA) and with hygromycin (to select for cells with the rtTA) and clones were picked. Exposure of some of those cell lines to doxycycline showed a constant decrease in PFM expression over a course of seven days. The results for clones H3-2-1 and H3-10 are shown in **Fig. 2.13**.

Fig. 2.13

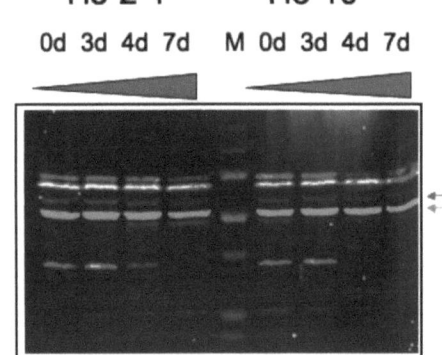

Fig. 2.13 Generation of U2OS cell lines, which inducibly downregulate PFM using the Tet-system. U2OS cell clones (H3-2-1, H3-10) showed a time dependent decrease in the PFM band (red, indicated by red arrow) in cells, which had been exposed to doxycycline for various time points (3d, 4d, 7d) compared to cells, which were not exposed (0d). The intensity of the tubulin band (green, indicated by green arrow) remained unchanged.
M: protein marker
d: days (of exposure to doxycycline)

Since neither the cell line that constitutively downregulated PFM nor the ones that inducibly downregulated PFM show an obvious phenotype (by gene expression or FACS profile), we decided to generate PFM knockout MEFs.

2.3 Knockout of Pfm in MEFs increases cell death and reduces the expression of genes involved in cell growth and proliferation

In a further attempt to generate cells with downregulated Pfm expression, we collaborated with the "Institut Clinique de la Souris", Illkirch, France (ICS), to create Pfm$^{fl/fl}$ mice. To this end, two loxP sites flanking exon 2 of Pfm were cloned into the genome of mouse ES cells. The Pfm$^{fl/wt}$ ES cells were genotyped by the ICS by southern blotting (data not shown) and Pfm$^{fl/wt}$ mice generated. The mice were crossed to produce Pfm$^{fl/fl}$ mice. MEFs from those mice were genotyped by PCR (**fig. 2.14**).

Fig. 2.14

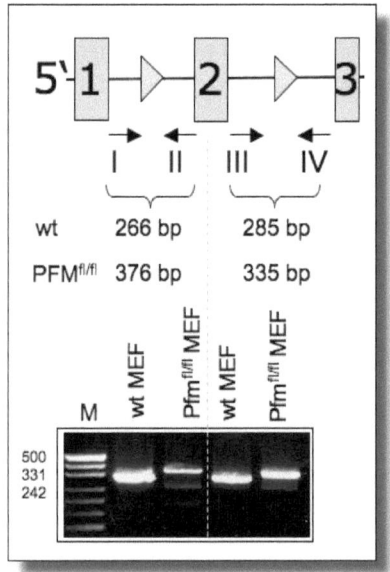

Fig. 2.14: Genomic DNA from Pfm$^{l/fl}$ and wt mice was extracted and genotyped by PCR. Four primers were designed (I, II, III, IV) and used to amplify regions that contained the two loxP sites. PCR products that contained a loxP site (from genetically modified mice) could be differentiated from DNA without a loxP site (from wt animals) by size (376bp and 335bp in contrast to 266bp and 285bp). The arrows indicate wether primers are forward or reverse. The numbers and the yellow squares represent the first three exons of the HRPT2 gene.
M: DNA marker

   Symbol for the two loxP-sites

Pfm$^{fl/fl}$ MEFs were prepared and infected with Adenovirus, encoding Cre-recombinase. Infected cells lost their Pfm gene, and thereby the expression of Pfm two to four days post infection. The decrease of Pfm expression in the primary MEF culture was monitored at the DNA level. Consequently, genomic DNA of infected and uninfected cells was isolated 3d after infection and analysed for deletion of Pfm exon 2. As shown in **Fig. 2.15** Pfm knockout cells were successfully generated and the two loxP-sites were functional.

Fig. 2.15

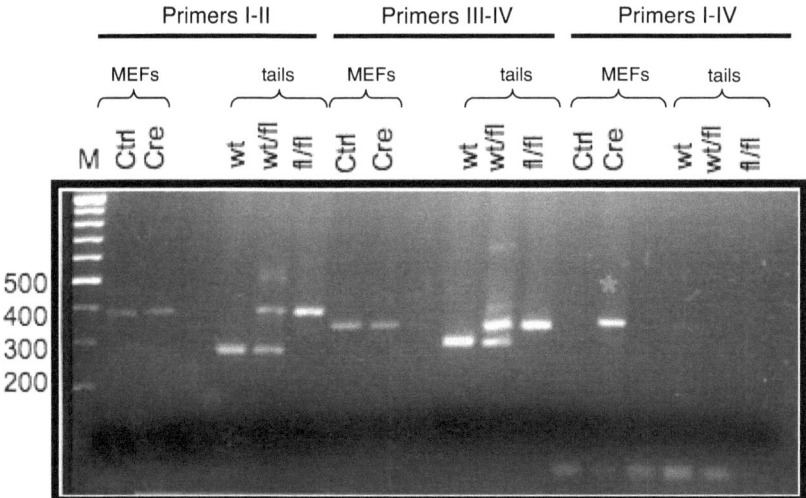

Fig. 2.15: The loxP sites of Pfm$^{fl/fl}$ MEFs loose exon 2 of the Pfm gene upon Cre expression. Genomic DNA of uninfected (Ctrl) and Cre-infected Pfm$^{fl/fl}$ MEFs was prepared and analysed by PCR with primers amplifying the 5'-loxP site, the 3'-loxP site and the whole floxed locus. As an additional control, tail DNA from wt, fl/fl, and from heterozygous (Pfm$^{fl/wt}$) animals was included. As expected, excision of exon 2 of HRPT2 was only detected in Cre-infected Pfm$^{fl/fl}$ MEFs (marked by the red asterix) but not in the not infected Pfm$^{fl/fl}$ MEFs or in tails of wt, herteozygous or Pfm$^{fl/fl}$ mice. This demonstrates functionality of the two loxP sites in Cre-infected Pfm$^{fl/fl}$ MEFs. The same primers were used as in **Fig. 2.14**.
M: DNA marker

In a next step, the decrease of Pfm expression upon Cre expression was monitored on the mRNA level by qRT-PCR as well as on the protein level by WB followed by immunodetection. **Fig. 2.16** shows that Pfm expression of infected Pfm$^{fl/fl}$ MEFs yielded approximately 80-90% knockout cells when compared to control uninfected cells (**fig. 2.16**).

Fig. 2.16

a)

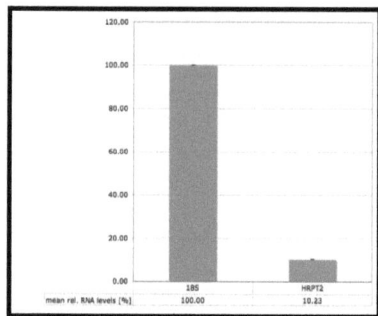

b)

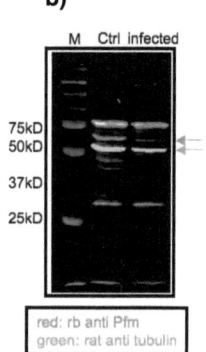

Fig. 2.16: Pfm expression can be knocked out in approximately 80-90% of all Adeno-Cre infected Pfm$^{fl/fl}$ MEFs. Pfm$^{fl/fl}$ MEFs were infected for 3d with Adeno-Cre. **a)** RNA of uninfected and infected Pfm$^{fl/fl}$ MEFs was isolated, reverse-transcribed into cDNA and analyzed by qRT-PCR. The mRNA levels of Pfm of infected Pfm$^{fl/fl}$ MEFs was reduced to approximately 10% of the Pfm mRNA of uninfected MEFs. The signal intensity was normalized using 18S rRNA. **b)** WCE of uninfected and infected Pfm$^{fl/fl}$ MEFs were prepared and separated by 10% PAGs, western blotted and immunodetected with antibodies against Pfm (red) and tubulin (green). The signal intensity of the specific Pfm band (indicated by red arrow) was dramatically reduced in infected Pfm$^{fl/fl}$ MEFs compared to Ctrl MEFs, while equal loading was confirmed by the tubulin band (indicated by green arrow).
M: protein marker

After infection, cells were splitted and further cultured. Interestingly, we observed that Adeno-Cre infected Pfm$^{fl/fl}$ MEFs showed enhanced cell death within 2-3d. This effect could be seen by morphological changes of the cells (**fig. 2.17a**) and was quantified by counting the cells using a hemocytometer (**fig. 2.17b**). In contrast to that, Adeno-Cre infected Pfm$^{wt/wt}$ MEFs showed no enhanced cell death (data not shown), confirming that the cell death observed was due to loss of Pfm and not due to the viral infection.

Fig. 2.17

a)

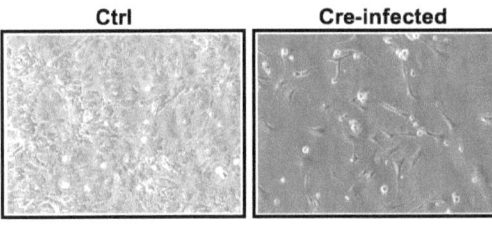

b)

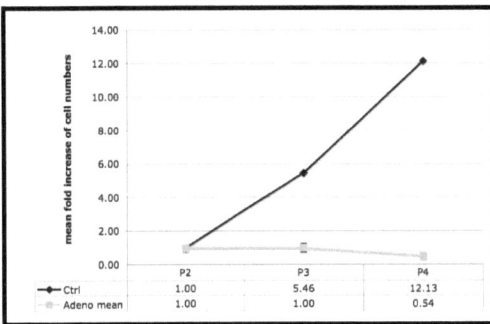

c)

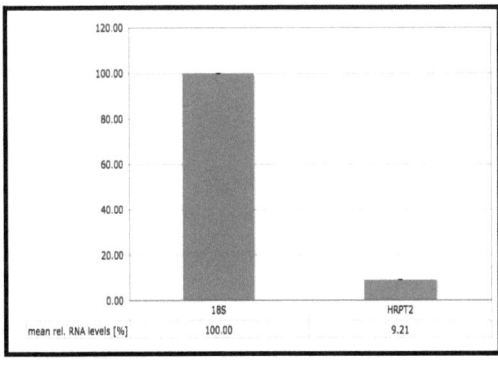

Fig. 2.17: Pfm$^{-/-}$ MEFs show enhanced cell death. Pfm$^{fl/fl}$ MEFs were infected for 3d with Adeno-Cre. **a)** Pictures of uninfected cells and of infected cells were taken. **b)** Cells were counted over a period of three passages. The numbers in the table reflect the number of cells counted using a hemocytometer. The results shown are the results of three independent experiments. **c)** As an additional control, RNA of uninfected and infected Pfm$^{fl/fl}$ MEFs was analyzed by qRT-PCR. The mRNA levels of PFM of infected Pfm$^{fl/fl}$ MEFs was reduced to 10% of the Pfm mRNA levels of uninfected MEFs (RNA of Pfm is labled as HRPT2). The signal intensity was normalized against 18S rRNA.

In a next step, we used qRT-PCR to analyze the MEFs for differences in mRNA expression of previously published target genes of Pfm and the hPaf1C (**fig. 2.18**). Igf1, Igf2, Hmg1 and Igfbp4 were all slightly downregulated to approximately 50-70% compared to control cells (**fig. 2.18**).

Fig. 2.18

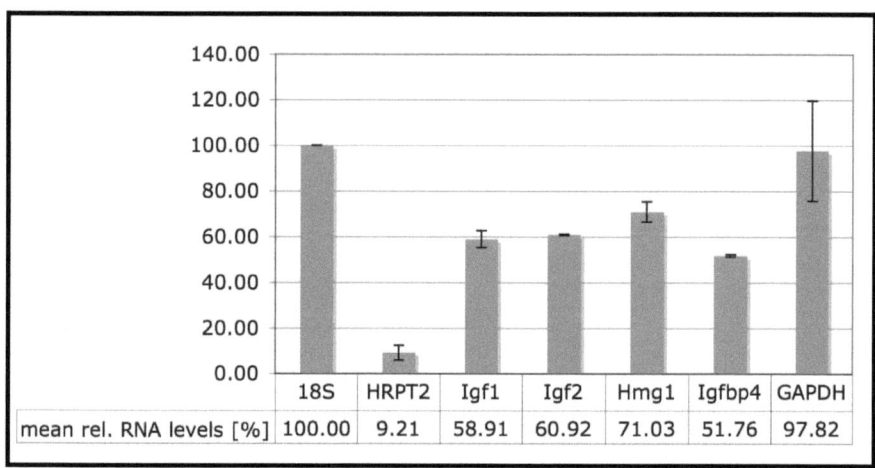

Fig. 2.18: Igf1, Igf2, Hmg1 and Igfbp4 but not Gapdh are downregulated upon Pfm knockout in MEFs. RNA of uninfected and Adeno-Cre infected Pfm$^{fl/fl}$ MEFs was analyzed by qRT-PCR. The mRNA levels of Pfm of Adeno-Cre infected Pfm$^{fl/fl}$ MEFs was reduced to approximately 10% of the Pfm mRNA levels of uninfected MEFs. Additionally, mRNA levels of previously published target genes Igf1, Igf2, Hmg1 and Igfbp4 were all downregulated to approximately 50-70% compared to uninfected MEFs. As an addititional control, cDNA levels of the housekeeping gene Gapdh were meassured. The Gapdh levels were unchanged. The signal intensity was normalized using 18S rRNA. Numbers in the table reflect the mean relative RNA levels from three independent experiments of Adeno-Cre infected Pfm$^{fl/fl}$ MEFs compared to uninfected Pfm$^{fl/fl}$ MEFs in %.
M: DNA marker

Upon binding to insulin, IGF-I, or IGFII receptor, IGF-I/II activates the PI3K-pathway, which controls apoptosis and cell proliferation and is frequently perturbed in various cancers. An active PI3K-pathway leads to an active AKT phosphorylated at Ser473 and Thr308, which in turn inactivates GSK3β by phosphorylating it at Ser9. In line with Wang et al. (2008), we show reduced IGF-I/II expression in Pfm$^{-/-}$ primary MEFs. Consequently, we were interested to find out if this reduced expression of IGF-I/II reduces the activity of the PI3K pathway and leads to lower levels of Phospho-GSK3β (Ser9). Therefore Ctrl Pfm$^{fl/fl}$ MEFs and Adeno-Cre infected Pfm$^{fl/fl}$ MEFs were analyzed for differences in Phospho-GSK3β (Ser9) levels (**fig. 2.19**). To our surprise and despite reduced levels of Pfm, Phospho-GSK3β (Ser9) levels remained unchanged in Pfm$^{-/-}$ MEFs. Tubulin staining confirmed equal loading (**fig. 2.19**).

Fig. 2.19

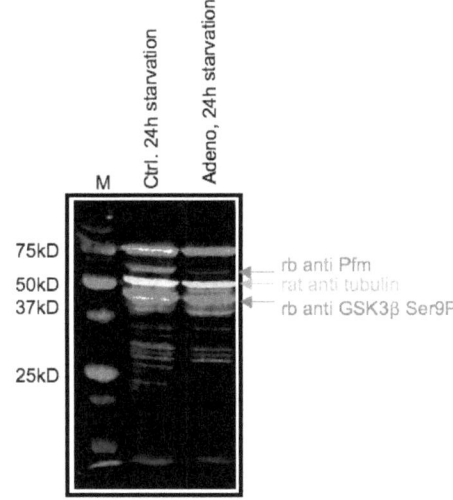

Fig. 2.19 Phospho-GSK3β (Ser9) levels are unaltered upon Pfm knockout in MEFs. PFM$^{fl/fl}$ MEFs were infected with Adeno-Cre virus. Cells were harvested, equal protein amounts of WCE per lane separated on a PAG, westernblotted and immunoblotted for Pfm (red, top arrow indicates the specific Pfm band), Tubulin (green, arrow indicates the specific tubulin band), and Phospho-GSK3β-Ser9 (red, lowest arrow indicates the specific Phospho-GSK3β-Ser9 band).
M: Marker
rb: rabbit

AKT is an upstream component of the PI3K-pathway and is activated by phosphorylation at Ser473 and Thr308 by PDK1 upon insulin or IGF-I/II binding to the IGF-I/II receptor. Since GSK3β Ser9P levels were not affected, we tested if its upstream kinase AKT is activated. Consequently, we analyzed the phosphorylation status of AKT after starvation by WB and immunodetection (**fig. 2.20**). While the intensity of the Pfm band was dramatically reduced in Pfm$^{-/-}$ MEFs, AKT-Phosphorylation levels and total AKT levels remained unaltered. Tubulin staining confirmed equal loading. Similar results were obtained for exponentially growing, non-starved cells.

Fig. 2.20

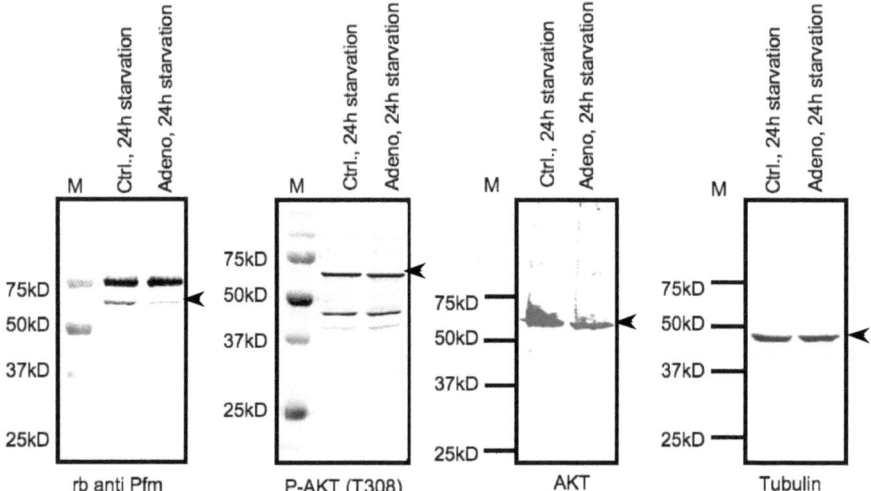

Fig. 2.20: Phosphorylation of AKT at Thr308 is unaltered in Pfm$^{-/-}$ MEFs. Pfm$^{fl/fl}$ MEFs were infected with Adeno-Cre virus and starved for 24h (normal growth medium without serum). Cells were harvested, equal protein amounts of WCE per lane separated on a PAG, westernblotted and immunodetected with the antibodies against PFM against Thr308-phosphorolated AKT, against AKT, and against tubulin. Arrow indicate the specific bands.
M: Marker

2.4 Generation of polyclonal antibodies against murine Pfm

Polyclonal antibodies are necessary tools to study the function of any protein. In collaboration with Eurogentec S.A., Seraign, Belgium we therefore generated two polyclonal antibodies against murine Pfm, one against the N-terminal part and one against the C-terminal part. Both of these antibodies are functional and have been tested in WB.

In a first step, the two halfs of murine Pfm were expressed in *E. coli* and purified on GSH beads. Three eluates for each half were loaded on a PAG, stained with Coomassie and visualized using the Odyssey system (**fig. 2.21**). The purified GST fusion proteins were sent to Eurogentec S.A., where the antibodies were produced in rabbits under standard conditions (100µg of antigen per rabbit and immmunization).

Fig. 2.21

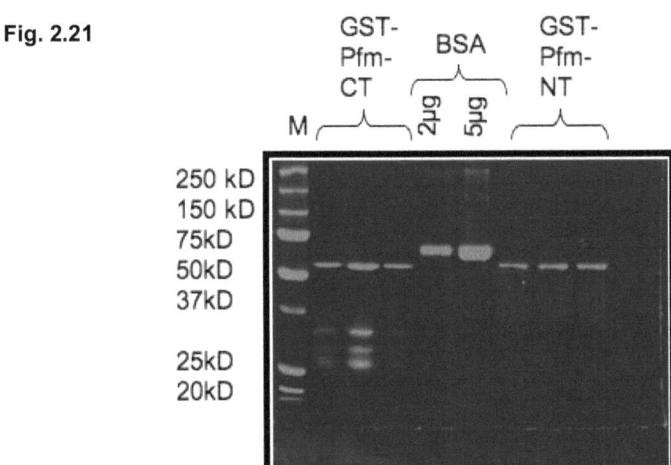

Fig. 2.21: Bacterial expression of GST-CT-Pfm and GST-NT-Pfm. The C- and the N-terminal part of Pfm were produced in *E. coli*, purified on GSH columns, separated on a PAG and visualized by Coomassie staining.
M: protein marker

(the two Pfm halfs were produced and purified by Bogdan Gerya and Felix Hauler)

The antibody sera sent by Eurogentec were affinity-purified on MBP-Pfm columns to enrich for antibodies recognizing Pfm. In a first test, the antibodies were used in immunodetection of bacterially expressed, purified and blotted GST-tagged versions of the N-terminal part and C-terminal part of Pfm and GST alone. As expected, the purified antibodies against the N-terminal part and the C-terminal part of Pfm both recognized GST-Pfm but not GST alone. (**fig. 2.22**).

Fig. 2.22

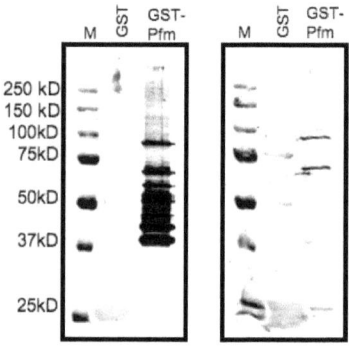

Fig. 2.22: The polyclonal antibodies against Pfm recognized bacterially expressed and purified GST-Pfm. Bacterially expressed and purified GST-Pfm and GST were separated on PAGs and western blotted. Both purified antibodies against the C- and the N-terminal part of Pfm specifically recognized GST-Pfm and not GST. The arrows indicate the expected sizes of the two GST-tagged halves of Pfm. M: protein marker

Finally, the two polyclonal antibodies were tested for their ability to specifically recognize endogenous murine Pfm in WB. For that, WCE of infected and uninfected Pfm$^{fl/fl}$ MEFs were used. Both antibodies detected a band at the expected size. Adeno-Cre infected Pfm$^{fl/fl}$ MEFs showed a dramatically reduced Pfm band, further confirming the specificity of the two antibodies generated (**fig. 2.23**).

Fig. 2.23

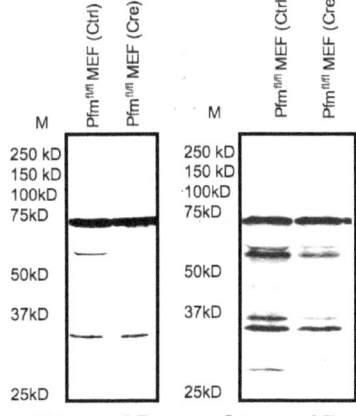

Fig. 2.23: The polyclonal antibodies against Pfm recognized endogenous murine Pfm. WCE of PFM$^{fl/fl}$ MEFs were separated on PAGs and western blotted. Both purified antibodies against the C- and the N-terminal part of Pfm gave specific bands at the expected size. Prior treatment of PFM$^{fl/fl}$ MEFs with Adeno-Cre virus prevented the appearance of this band, confirming the specificity of the two antibodies.
M: protein marker

3 Discussion

3.1 The Paf1 complex (hPaf1C) is a dense network of interactions between its five components

To identify the molecular architecture of the hPaf1C, we cloned the five human Paf1C components and URI into baculo transfer vectors, produced the respective baculoviruses and expressed URI and the hPaf1C components as GST-tagged fusion proteins in *Sf9* cells. The amounts of purified proteins were then equilibrated and tested for their ability to pull down radioactively labeled *in vitro* translated, untagged hPaf1C components and URI. In our analyses, every possible combination of direct interactions within the hPaf1C was tested (i.e. every hPaf1C component was *in vitro* translated and tested for direct interaction with any other GST-tagged hPaf1C members expressed in *Sf9* cells). We found that the hPaf1C is a dense network of direct interactions among its components Paf1, PFM, Ctr9, Ski8 and Leo1 (**fig. 2.2** and **fig 2.5**). Leo1 is the only component that associates with only one partner, Paf1. The other four members of the hPaf1C each bind to one another. We therefore suggest that the molecular architecture of the hPaf1C consists of a core hPaf1C that comprises PFM, Ski8, Ctr9 and Paf1 and of an auxiliary hPaf1C that contains Leo1. Since all direct interactions between two Paf1C components were observed in the absence of any of the other three members, it seems unlikely that the loss of one component (f.e. PFM) would affect the direct interaction between the other Paf1C components. Apart from that, we found that GST-PFM pulls down *in vitro* translated PFM, demonstrating that PFM is able to form homodimers and possibly homo-multimers (**fig. 2.3**). Finally, we were able to show that the unconventional prefoldin RPB5 interactor (URI) interacts directly with PFM but not with any other hPaf1C component (**fig. 2.4**). URI is also known as RBP5-mediating protein (RMP) and has been initially described as a novel RBP5 interacting protein (Dorjsuren, et al. 1998). Interestingly, URI has been shown to inhibit PP1γ, thereby being an important component of a homeostatic signaling mechanism involved in setting the mitochondrial threshold for apoptosis in accord with growth factor and nutritional signals (Djouder, et al. 2007).

Those first results of our interaction studies yieled a model that summarizes the *in vitro* interactions found (**fig. 2.5**). Interestingly, an interaction between Ski8 on the one hand and Paf1 or PFM on the other was only observed when Paf1 or PFM were *in vitro* translated and Ski8 expressed as a GST fusion protein. This interaction however was never observed *vice versa* (*in vitro* translated Ski8 was never pulled down by PFM or Paf1). There are two likely explanations for this finding. Firstly, in contrast to IVT or bacterial expression systems, the baculo system allows for post translational modifications to occur. The lacking interaction between *in vitro* translated Ski8 and *Sf9* cell expressed hPaf1 or PFM could therefore be explained if those post translational modifications on hSki8 were required for the interaction with hPaf1 and PFM. Secondly and more likely, it could be that the GST at the N-terminal part of Paf1 and PFM structurally prevents Ski8 from binding to PFM or hPaf1. Indeed, our later findings with truncated hPaf1 and PFM actually show that Ski8 binds to the N-terminal part of hPaf1, further supporting this hypothesis at least for the interaction between hPaf1 and Ski8. Due to tertiary and quaternary structures of proteins, the later finding that Ski8 binds a domain that is located almost in the central part of the primary structure of PFM, does not exclude that the GST at the N-terminal part of PFM prevents the interaction between *in vitro* translated Ski8 and GST-PFM.

Next, we were interested to see if any of the six naturally occuring, clinically relevant point mutations of PFM affect the ability of PFM to directly interact with members of the hPaf1C. Since the most N-terminal PFM point mutation, PFM M1L, is a point mutation in the start codon that prevents translation of the whole protein, it was not considered in our analysis. Consequently, we generated five different PFM point mutants and produced the following radioactively labeled *in vitro* translates: K34Q, L64P, R292K, D379N. None of the PFM point mutants exhibited any defect in binding to Paf1, Ski8, Ctr9, PFM or URI (**fig. 2.6**) suggesting that the molecular architecture of the hPaf1C is intact in patients expressing those PFM point mutations. Our findings are especially interesting, since this is to our knowledge the first study on the binding characteristics of PFM point mutants. Apart from the binding function of PFM, other - yet to be discovered- tumour suppressor functions of PFM are consequently impaired in those PFM point mutants.

Obviously, more dramatic PFM mutations were needed to disrupt binding to members of the hPaf1C. For that reason we continued our experiments with one of

3 Discussion

the largest naturally occuring and clinically relevant PFM truncation, PFM R222X. Most of the currently known PFM mutations lead to N-terminally truncated versions of PFM that are shorter than 222 aa (Wang et al. 2005) (i.e. shorter than PFM R222X), suggesting that the main tumour suppressor functions of PFM are located at the more C-terminal part (aa 222-531) of the protein. At the same time, the functions of the first 222 aa of PFM still remain to be discovered. In an attempt to understand if the abilities of N-terminally truncated PFM versions to bind members of the hPaf1C are affected by the truncations, we used PFM R222X in our binding assay. Despite the fact that almost half of the protein was still expressed, none of the hPaf1C components or URI was able to bind to it (**fig. 2.7**). These data suggest that the region C-terminally of 222 aa is used to bind to any member of the hPaf1C. Since this region overlaps with the part of PFM lost in hyperplasia, our findings further link the tumour suppressor function of PFM to its ability to interact with the hPaf1C.

To increase the resolution of our model of the molecular architecture of the hPaf1C, we *in vitro* translated the C- and N-terminal halfs of Paf1, Ctr9 and PFM and tested them in our binding assay. An overview of the precise length of each half is shown in **Fig. 3.1**.

The results from these experiments (**fig. 2.8, fig. 2.9**, and **fig. 2.10**) form the basis for our model of the molecular architecture of the hPaf1C (**fig. 2.11**). According to our data, the N-terminal halfs seem to be the main sites of protein interaction within the hPaf1C. This holds true for any interaction observed, except for the interaction between PFM and Ctr9, as our data suggest that PFM binds Ctr9 at least twice, once at the C-terminal part and once at the N-terminal part of Ctr9. Ctr9 contains a total number of nine tetratricopeptide repeats (TPRs) dispersed over the whole protein. TPRs are 34 aa long repeat motifs typically involved in protein-protein interactions (Cortajarena and Regan 2006; D'Andrea and Regan 2003; Hirano, et al. 1990; Lamb, et al. 1995). It can be speculated that those TPR motifs within Ctr9 mediate the interaction between PFM and Ctr9.

In detail, our results show that the N-terminal half of PFM (aa 1-270) is mediating the interaction to hPaf1 and hSki8. Since we could show in our previous findings that PFM R222X, does not bind to any hPaf1 *in vitro* (**fig. 2.7**), we propose that aa 223-270 of PFM constitute the domain responsible for mediating the interaction of PFM to hPaf1 and hSki8 (**fig. 2.11**). These results are consistent with previous reports, which claimed that hPaf1C components interact with a PFM region located C-terminally of aa 218 (Rozenblatt-Rosen et al. 2005; Yart et al. 2005).

Fig. 3.1

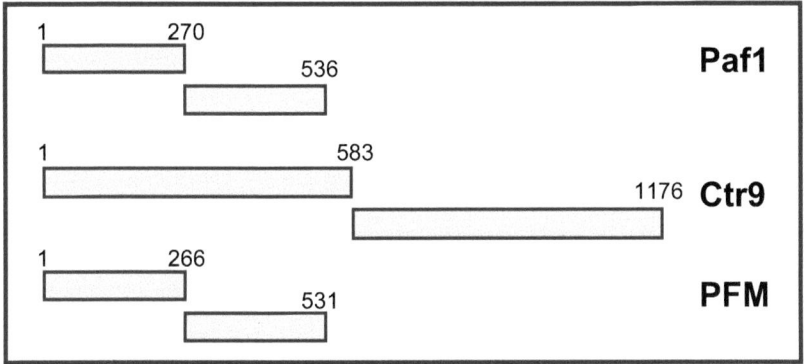

Fig. 3.1: Overview of the C- and N-terminal halfs of hPaf1C expressed as *in vitro* translates to map regions of direct protein-protein interactions between hPaf1C. Each protein was expressed in two halfs of roughly the same size. Numbers on top of each protein half represent the aa number.

The location of the Paf1/Ski8 Binding Domain (PSBD) is visualized in **Fig. 3.2**. Surprisingly, this domain is almost identical to the β-catenin interaction domain. The region with which PFM interacts with URI and Ctr9 is not marked in this figure. However, we know from our experiements that PFM R222X does neither bind to URI nor Ctr9 and we can therefore conclude that PFM uses a region located C-terminally of aa 222 to interact with URI and with Ctr9. From these data, we cannot exclude that the PSBD is also mediating this interaction between PFM on the one side and Ctr9 as well as URI on the other.

Fig. 3.2

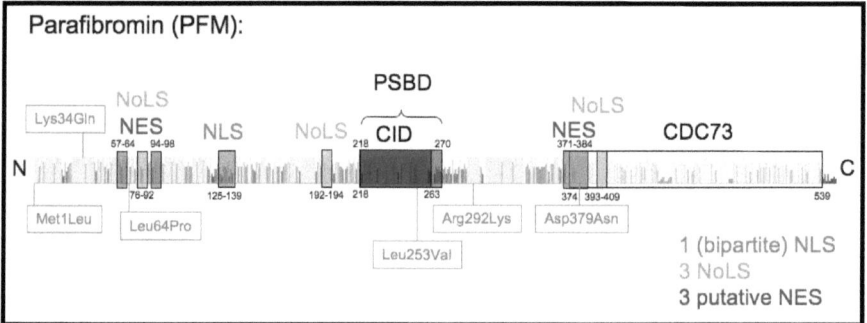

Fig. 3.2: The PSBD is located in the center of PFM and overlaps with the CID. A yellow line represents each amino acid (aa) of parafibromin. The longer the line and the more yellow, the more conserved is the respective amino acid among the different species. Several functional domains on PFM have been defined so far (one bipartite NLS, three putative NES, three NoLS, the CID and the CDC73 domain). Here, we report the finding of a new domain that is mediating the interaction to Paf1 and Ski8. The locations of the six clinically relevant PFM point mutations that are currently known are also shown in the figure. The six species used for the homology search were: *Homo sapiens*, *Mus musculus*, *Rattus norvegicus*, *Bos taurus*, *Drosophila melanogaster*, *Caenorhabditis elegans*, and *Xenopus laevi*.
N: N-terminus
C: C-terminus

This is the first systematic study on the direct interactions within the hPaf1C. However, there has been one report on the direct interaction within the yPaf1C (Schwahn 2007). Based on their results from IP experiments with yeast strains mutant for combinations of yPaf1C components, the authors drew a model of direct interactions within the yPaf1C that summarizes their findings (**fig.3.3**).

Fig. 3.3

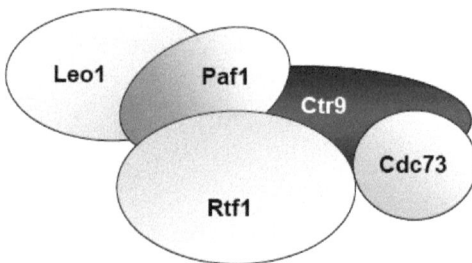

Fig. 3.3: Model summarizing the direct interactions within the yPaf1C. The core of the yPaf1C is made up by Paf1 and Ctr9, that interact with each other and with Rtf1. In addition, each of them also interacts with either Cdc73 or Leo1. Cdc73 stablizes the contact between Rtf1 on the one hand and Ctr9 and Paf1 on the other (taken from Schwahn, 2007).

Interestingly, the two Paf1C models share several similarities. In both cases, Ctr9 and Paf1 are located at the core of the complex, with direct interations to each other and to all of the remaining members of the complex. Similar to our findings for the hPaf1C, Schwahn et al. found that Paf1 binds to the N-terminal part of Ctr9 (Schwahn 2007). Furthermore, the only binding partner of Leo1 is in both cases Paf1. In addition, the direct interaction between Cdc73 and Ctr9 was also observed with the human homologues (C-terminal-PFM binding to the C-terminal part and N-terminal part of Ctr9). In comparison to Cdc73 however, PFM is much better integrated into the Paf1C, since PFM does not only directly bind to Ctr9 (as Cdc73 does in the yPaf1C) but also to Paf1 and Ski8 (N-terminal part of Paf1 and Ski8 bind PSBD). A recent study confirmed some of the data from Schwan by demonstrating that loss of Cdc73 or Rtf1 reduces the association of the yPaf1C with RNAPII, but does not disrupt interactions between the remaining yPaf1C components (Nordick et al. 2008). Finally, Ski8, which is not part of yPaf1C, has three direct binding partners (PFM at PSBD, Paf1- N-terminal part, and Ctr9- N-terminal part) within the hPaf1C, while yRtf1 directly bound only to yCtr9 and yPaf1.

3.2 Generation of human cancer cell lines that inducibly and constitutively downregulate PFM

In order to identify cell biological functions of PFM, we generated HeLa cells, which constitutively downregulate hPaf1C components on the mRNA and protein level (**fig. 2.12**). To our surprise, we did not see any phenotype neither if PFM nor if any other Paf1C component was downregulated. We repeated those experiments with other cell lines (786-0, RPE-1) and obtained the same results. In order to exclude adaptation of the cell lines to PFM downregulation, we used the same hairpins and the Tet system to generate U2OS cells, that downregulate PFM inducibly upon exposure of doxycycline for up to 7d (**fig. 2.13**). These cell lines showed a time-dependent downregulation of PFM upon addition of doxycline to the medium. Once again however, no consequences on morphology or cell cycle (measured by FACS analysis) were observed. While effects of PFM on the morphology have not been investigated so far, we were surprised that the PFM knockdown cells appeared to cycle normally. This finding is in contrast to the previous reports that PFM knockdown by siRNA in

HeLa cells increases the fraction of cells in S-Phase (Yart et al. 2005) and PFM overexpression in HeLa, HEK293 and NIH-3T3 cells blocks the cell cycle in G1 (Iwata et al. 2007; Zhang et al. 2006). There are three possible reasons why the results of our studies differe from the results in literature. Firstly, the cell lines used in our study (HeLa, 786-O, RPE-1 and U2OS) are not fully congruent with the cell lines used in other studies where the effects of PFM on the cell type were reported. Secondly and in contrast to some of the other studies, we downregulated PFM instead of overexpressing it and finally, we used a retroviral system instead of siRNA to downregulate PFM. Since transfection of siRNA is more toxic than retroviral vectors, it might explain the cell death seen in those studies. Apart from that, it could of course also be that the antibiotic selection for shRNA for 5d-7d in our retroviral system used gave the cells enough time to adapt to reduced levels of PFM.

Apart from all that, our later results show that Pfm knockout causes cell death in MEFs (**fig. 2.17**). This phenotype was not observed in any of our cell lines that downregulated PFM constitutively or inducible. There are two main reasons that can explain this. Firstly, infecting Pfm$^{fl/fl}$ MEFs with Adeno-Cre reduced Pfm expression in infected cells much more dramatically than in cell lines, which downregulate parafibromin. The different basal expression levels of parafibromin in the three systems used could possible explain different phenotypes. The second explanation is based on the argument that all cell lines that constitutively downregulated PFM were selected for at least 5d with puromycine while PFM was downregulated. In addition, even the inducible cell lines showed a clear downregulation of PFM only after seven days of doxycycline exposure. During those periods, the cells have the time to adapt to the slowly downregulated PFM, thereby masking the increased level of cell death.

3.3 Knockout of Pfm in MEFs increases cell death and reduces the expression of genes involved in cell growth and proliferation

To identify cellular functions of Pfm, we decided to change the system and create Pfm knockout MEFs by firstly generating Pfm$^{fl/fl}$ mice, secondly isolating Pfm$^{fl/fl}$ MEFs and finally infecting those MEFs with adenovirus harbouring a Cre expression cassette (Adeno-Cre). In collaboration with "Institut Clinique de la Souris", we generated Pfm$^{fl/fl}$ mice and confirmed their genotype by southern blotting and PCR (**fig. 2.14**). Adeno-Cre infected isolated Pfm$^{fl/fl}$ MEFs showed a knockout of the Pfm gene on the genomic level (**fig. 2.15**) and downregulation of Pfm on the mRNA and protein level (**fig. 2.16**). Pfm$^{fl/fl}$ MEFs, which had been infected with Adeno-Cre underwent cell death approximately 2-3d after infection as shown by reduced cell numbers (**fig 2.17**). This finding is coherent with the results of Wang et al who claimed that primary Pfm$^{-/-}$ MEFs undergo apoptosis (Wang et al. 2008). It seems however to contradict another study that showed that Pfm downregulation in MEFs reduces the number of apoptotic cells (Lin et al. 2007). The differences between our results and the findings of Lin et al. may be explained by the fact that we used primary, whereas Lin et al used immortalized MEFs (NIH-3T3 cells).

In a next step, we analyzed the cells for differences in gene expression by qRT-PCR. Our results show a modest reduction (to approximately 50-70% of wt leves) of the expression of the known Pfm target genes Igf1, Igf2, Hmg1, and Igfbp4 but not of the control genes 18S rRNA and Gapdh (**fig. 2.18**). These results are in agreement with the only other report on this subject (Wang et al. 2008). IgfI/II are the extracellular ligands of the PI3K-pathway, which is known to positively regulate cell survival, cell growth, metabolism and proliferation. Accordingly, components of this pathway are frequently mutated in different cancers. The lower levels of the extracellular ligands Igf-I/II in Pfm$^{-/-}$ MEFs suggest that Pfm positively regulates the PI3K-pathway. Such a positive role for Pfm in PI3K-signalling is likely independent of Pfm's function as a tumour supressor. Since activated Akt causes a cascade of phosphorylation events that result in the inactivation of key proteins (Bcl-2 antagonist of cell death, caspase 9, and forkhead transcription factor family) involved in apoptosis (Burgering and Kops 2002; Velcheti and Govindan 2006), reduced levels of activated Akt upon Pfm loss could however explain the increased levels of cell death in Pfm$^{-/-}$ MEFs. Very interesting is also the finding that Igfbp4 mRNA is downregulated upon Pfm loss, as Igfbp4 has recently been shown to inhibit canonical Wnt signalling independently of its Igf-binding activity (Zhu, et al. 2008). In contrast to a positive role of Pfm in Wnt signalling (Mosimann et al. 2006), this could represent an additional mechanism by which Pfm negatively regulates Wnt signalling.

Binding of the extracellular ligands IGF-I/II and insulin to their receptors activates the PI3K pathway that leads to the phosphorylation of AKT at Ser473 and Thr308 by PDK1 and to the inhibitory phosphorylation of GSK3β at Ser9 by AKT. To test the hypothesis that the activity of the PI3K pathway is reduced upon Pfm loss, we analyzed the phosphorylation status of GSK3β at Ser9 (**fig. 2.19**) and of AKT at Thr308 in serum starved cells in WB (**fig. 2.20**). Interestingly, neither Phospho-GSK3β (Ser9) nor Phospho-AKT (Thr308) was altered in Adeno-Cre infected Pfm$^{fl/fl}$ MEFs, showing that the PI3K pathway is not activated by the loss of Pfm in primary MEFs.

Several arguments can be brought forward to explain why no inactivation of the PI3K-pathway was observed upon Pfm knockout in MEFs. First of all, in order for Igf-I/II to activate the PI3K-pathway in thw wild type setting, it must be secreted as they bind to extracellular Insulin-, Igf-I-, or Igf-II (and possibly other) receptors. In our hypothesis, that the PI3K pathway is inactivated upon PFM loss (since Igf-I/II is expression reduced upon PFM loss) we consequently assume that Igf-I/II are secreted and activate the PI3K pathways of the MEFs in an autocrine or paracrine fashion. We have no evidence that this first precondition is actually met in our experiments. Apart from that, our data show that Igfbp4 is also downregulated in Pfm$^{-/-}$ MEFs. IGFBP4 binds to both IGF-I and IGF-II and has been shown to be a positive and negative regulator of IGF signalling (Baxter 2000; Firth and Baxter 2002; Mohan and Baylink 2002; Ning, et al. 2008; Rajaram, et al. 1997; Sitar, et al. 2006). Recent *in vitro* and *in vivo* studies demonstrated that IGFBP4 is exclusively inhibitory to IGF-II actions and suggested to function as a local reservoir of IGF-II actions (Ning et al. 2008). A second explanation why the PI3K-pathway is not inactivated upon Pfm knockout in primary MEFs could therefore be that Igfbp4 as well as potentially other inhibitors of IGF signalling are concomitantly downregulated upon Pfm loss. This could adjust the downregulated amounts of IgfI/II. Moreover, we know that Igf-I/II are only downregulated on the mRNA level, and can therefore not exclude that the relative protein levels of Igf-I/II and Igfbp4 are still higher. This is especially relevant since the mRNA levels were only mildly downregulated to 50-70% of wt levels and since the half-lives of Igf-I/II are in turn modulated by IGFBPs (Rajaram et al. 1997).

3.4 Generation of polyclonal antibodies against murine Pfm

In collaboration with the company AMS-Bio, we tried in the past to produce mouse monoclonal antibodies against Pfm. The supernatants of subclones were screened and despite initial encouraging results, none of the attempts to produce monoclonal antibodies against Pfm were successful (data not shown).

Consequently, we generated rabbit polyclonal antibodies against murine Pfm, one against the N-terminal part and one against the C-terminal part. Consequently, we expressed the N- and C-terminal part of Pfm (murine and human Pfm are identical) in *E. coli*, purified them with affinity chromatography on GSH beads, loaded them on PAGs, and visualized the protein staining with Coomassie (**fig. 2.21**). Both of the affinity-purified antibodies were tested in WB and both specifically recognized bacterially expressed and purified GST-Pfm (**fig. 2.22**) as well as endogenous murine Pfm (**fig. 2.23**). The antibodies yielded additional bands at approximately 75kD and at 30kD and the C-terminal-AB above that a further band at approximately 60kD. To our knowledge the N-terminal-AB is the first antibody described in the literature that recognizes exclusively the N-terminal part of Pfm.

4 Material and Methods

Part I: Material

4.1 General Chemicals and Material

Chemical/ Material	Provider
Acrylamide:bisacrylamide (29:1) (%w/v)	Bio-Rad
Agarose	Invitrogen
Amylose beads	New England Biolaboratories
10% APS (Ammonium Persulfate) (not older than two weeks)	SIGMA-Aldrich
Bacto tryptone	BD Biosciences
Bacto yeast extract	BD Biosciences
Borax	Merck
Boric Acid	Merck
Bradford Solution (Biorad-Protein Assay)	Bio-Rad
$CaCl_2$	SIGMA-Aldrich
Cloning discs (3mm, sterile, γ-irradiated)	SIGMA-Aldrich
Coomassie Brilliant Blue G250	Fluka
Coumaric Acid	Fluka
DEPC	SIGMA-Aldrich
DMP	SIGMA-Aldrich
Deoxyribonuclease I	SIGMA-Aldrich (from bovine panreas)
dNTPs	Fermentas
DTT	Axon lab
EDTA	Axon lab
1xEN3HANCE-Autoradiography Enhancer	Perkin Elmer
Ethanol	Merck
Ethanolamine	Fluka

Ethidium Bromide	Fluka
Fuji RX Films	Fuji
Glucose	Fluka
glutathione	SIGMA-Aldrich
Glutathion Sepharose 4B	GE Healthcare
99% Glycerole	Axon lab
Glycine	Fluka
98% H_2O_2	SIGMA-Aldrich
37% HCl	Fluka
HEPES	SIGMA-Aldrich
Isopropyl-1-thio-b-D-galactoside (IPTG), filter sterilized	Axon lab
K_2HPO_4	Merck
KCl	Fluka
Kodak Biomax MR Film	Kodak Biomax
KOH	Merck
LiCl	Fluka
Luminol (3-Aminophtalhydrazide)	Fluka
β-mercaptoethanol	Fluka
methanol	Merck
$MgCl_2$	Fluka
$MnCl_2$	Fluka
NaCitrate pH 7.5	Fluka
NaCl	Merck
NaF	Fluka
Na-HEPES pH 7.05	SIGMA-Aldrich
$Na_2HPO_4 \times 2H_2O$	Fluka
Nalgene 0.45µm PES membrane (0.45µm cellulose acetate syringe filter)	Semadeni
NaN_3	Fluka
NaOH	Merck
Nitrocellulose	Schleicher & Schuell
nonfat dried milk	Migros

Nonidet P40	Fluka
Oligofectamin Reagent	Invitrogen
PBS	Biochrom AG
Phenol:Chloroform 5:1	SIGMA-Aldrich
ortho-phosphoric acid	Merck
random hexamers	Promega and of Invitrogen
RNASIN	Promega
SDS	Fluka
SDS- polyacrylamide gel electrophoresis system	Hoefer
SYBR Green	Roche
TEMED (N,N,N',N'-tetramethylethylene diamine)	Fluka
Triethanolamine pH 11.5	SIGMA-Aldrich
Tris	SIGMA-Aldrich
Triton X-100	Fluka
Trizma	SIGMA-Aldrich
Tween-20	Riedel-de-Häen

4.2 Chemicals and Media used in Tissue Culture Experiments

Medium/ Chemical	Provider
ampicilin	Axon lab
β-mercaptoethanol	Fluka
BaculoGold DNA	BD Biosciences
chloramphenicol	Axon lab
doxycycline	SIGMA-Aldrich
DMEM	Gibco
DMSO	Fluka
doxycycline	SIGMA-Aldrich
FUGENE	Roche
G418 (neomycin)	Gibco

Grace's Insect Medium	Gibco
Hygromycine	Calbiochem
kanamycin	Axon lab
LB-Agar	BD Biosciences
LB medium	BD Biosciences
L-Glutamin	Gibco
PBS	Biochrome AG
Penicillin/ Streptomycin	Gibco
Polybrene (Hexadimethine Bromide)	SIGMA-Aldrich
puromycin	SIGMA-Aldrich
Trypan Blue	Gibco
Trypsin	Gibco

4.3 Antibodies

Antigen	Origin raised in	Company	Application	Dilution	Polyclonal/ monoclonal
GST	rabbit	SIGMA	WB	1:2000	p
Tubulin	rat	Harlan Sera Lab, YL1/2,	WB	1:1500	m
Parafibromin	rabbit	Self-made by AY with GST-C-term (378-531)	WB	1:500	p
Parafibromin	rabbit	Self-made by AY (cloning), FH and FK with GST-C-term (270-531)	WB	1:250	p
Parafibromin	rabbit	Self-made by AY (cloning), BG and FK with GST-N-term (2-270)	WB	1:250	p
p27	rabbit	Santa Cruz sc-528	WB	1:100	p
p21	goat	Santa Cruz sc-397-G	WB	1;100	p
Phospho-GSK3β (Ser9)	rabbit	Cell Signalling	WB	1:500, BSA	p

Phospho-AKT (Thr308)	rabbit	9295 Santa Cruz, Sc-16646	WB	1:500, BSA	p
Phospho-AKT (Ser473)	rabbit	Cell Signalling 4058	WB	1:1000, BSA	p
Secondaries					
Rat IgG	goat	Rockland	WB	1:2000	p, IRDye™800-linked
Rabbit IgG	rabbit	Rockland	WB	1:2000	p, IRDye™600-linked
Rabbit IgG	rabbit	Rockland	WB	1:2000	p, IRDye™800-linked
Mouse IgG	goat	Rockland	WB	1:2000	p, IRDye™600-linked
Mouse IgG	goat	Rockland	WB	1:2000	p, IRDye™800-linked
Goat IgG	donkey	Rockland	WB	1:2000	p, IRDye™800-linked
Rabbit IgG	donkey	GE Healthcare	WB	1:1000	p, HRP-linked
Mouse IgG	sheep	GE Healthcare	WB	1:1000	p, HRP-linked

4.4 Restriction Enzymes

All restriction enzyme were purchased from Roche or New England Biolaboratories and were used according to the suppliers recommendations.

4.5 Radiochemicals

For all in vitro translation experiementes, 1mCi of 35L-Methionine with a radioactive concentration of 10mCi/mL and a specific activity of 1175Ci/mmol from GE Healthcare was used.

4.6 Length standards (for proteins and DNA)

Number	Name	Fragments
1	Precision Plus Protein™ Standards (Bio-Rad)	10kD, 15kD, 20kD, 25kD, 37kD, 50kD, 75kD, 100kD, 150kD, 250kD
2	GeneRuler™ 100bp DNA Ladder Plus (NEB)	100bp, 200bp, 300bp, 400bp, 500bp, 600bp, 700bp, 800bp, 900bp, 1031bp, 1200bp, 1500bp, 2000bp, 3000bp
3	1kb DNA ladder (NEB)	0.5kbp, 1kbp, 1.5kbp, 2kbp, 3kbp, 4kbp, 5kbp, 6kbp, 8kbp, 10kbp
4	DNA marker pUc19 V (US Biological)	67bp, 110/111bp, 147bp, 190bp, 242bp, 331bp, 404bp, 489/501bp
5	DNA marker III (Roche Diagnostics)	564bp, 831bp, 947bp, 1375bp, 1584bp, 1904bp, 2027bp, 3530bp, 4268bp, 4973bp, 5148bp, 21226bp

4.7 DNA Oligonucleotides

Except for oligonucleotides for antisense experiments, oligonucleotides were ordered from Microsynth (genomics scale, lyophilized, desalted).

4.7.1 Oligonucleotides for Sequencing

Number	Name	Target	Sequence
1	TMPseq2466	TMP	GCGCGAAGGGGCCACCAAAGA
2		LMP	GCCTCGATCCTCCCTTTATC
3	pfm M340X	pMal-c2-PFM2-531	GCATGGATCCGCGGACGTGCTTAGCG
4	P529E	pMal-c2-PFM2-531	GCATGAATTCTGTCAGTGGAAAAAATTGC
5	pfmhs GST P1135E	pMal-c2-PFM2-531	CGATCTCGAGTCAGAATCTCAAGTGCG
6	P1Ctr9	Ctr9 constructs	GGGTTAGTACGCAATGCTTTCT
7	P2Ctr9	Ctr9 constructs	AAGGGCCATTTGAAGAAGGTC
8	P3Ctr9	Ctr9 constructs	CATCGGGATACTGTTCTGTGACCT
9	P4Ctr9	Ctr9 constructs	TCGTGCTCTGGCCATCTACAAACA
10	P5Ctr9	Ctr9 constructs	TTTGATTTGGCCCTTGCTGCTACA
11	P6Ctr9	Ctr9 constructs	CCATCAATGAAGGGAAAAATAAA
12	P1Leo1	Leo1 constructs	CGAAACTCACCTTCAGACCTC
13	P2Leo1	Leo1 constructs	CGACCAGCCATTGGCAAGAT
14	P3Leo1	Leo1 constructs	GAGGACGAGGGAGCTTCACATC
15	P4Leo1	Leo1 constructs	TTTATCTTCTCTGCCCCATTTTC
16	P1.pAcGST	pAcGHLT-A	ATACGCCGGACCAGTGAACAGAGG

| 17 | pAcGHLTA24 65 | pAcGHLT-A | AAGAGCGTGCAGAGATTT |

4.7.2 Oligonucleotides for Cloning

*numbers represent bp number

Number	Name	Sequence (5'->3')	Construct to be cloned
1	HRPT2for1	ATATGAATTCGCGGACGTGCTTAGCG	pMal-c2-PFM2-531 (SalI/EcoRI)
2	HRPT2rev2right	CGGACGGACGGAAAGCTTTCAGAATCTCAAGTGCG	
3	forSki8EcoRI	ATTAATTAGAATTCATGACCAACCAGTACG	pcDNA3-Ski8 (EcoRI/XhoI)
4	revSki8XhoI	ATTAATTACTCGAGTTAAATTGGACAATCA	
5	forP1	ATTAATTAGGAGCTCGCGCCCACCATCCAGA	pAcGHLT-A-Paf1 (SacI/KpnI)
6	revP1	ATTAGGTACCTCAATCACTGTCACTG	
7	forH1	ATTAATTAGGAGCTCGCGGACGTGCTTAGCG	pAcGHLT-A-Parafibromin (SacI/KpnI)
8	revH1	ATTAGGTACCTCAGAATCTCAAGTGC	
9	forS1	ATTAATTAGGAGCTCACCAACCAGTACGGTA	pAcGHLT-A-Ski8 (SacI/KpnI)
10	revS1	ATTAGGTACCTTAAATTGGACAATCA	
11	forL1	ATTAATTAGGAGCTCGCGGATATGGAGGATC	pAcGHLT-A-Leo1 (SacI/KpnI)
12	revL1	ATTAGGTACCTCAATCATCATCTTCCT	
13	Ctr9hforNotI	ATTAATTAATGCGGCCGCATCGCGGGGCTCCATCG	pAcGHLT-A-Ctr9 (NotI/PstI)
14	Ctr9hrevPstI	ATTACTGCAGCTAGTCACTATCATCT	
15	forCtr9KpnI	ATTAATTAGGTACCATGTCGCGGGGCTCCATC	pCMV-XL5-Ctr91-1749* (KpnI/XhoI)
16	revCtr91749XhoI	ATTAATTACTCGAGTCAAGGACCCCATTCTTGTTT	
17	forCtr91749KpnI	ATTAATTAGGTACCATGGGTCAGAAGAAGTTT	pCMV-XL5-Ctr911749-3522* (XhoI/KpnI)
18	revCtr9XhoI	ATTAATTACTCGAGCTAGTCGCTATCATCTGA	
19	forHRPT2EcoRI	ATTAATTAGAATTCATGGCGGACGTGCTTA	pcDNA3-PFML253V
20	revHRPT2XhoI	ATTAATTACTCGAGTCAGAATCTCAAGTGC	
21	forHRPT2Leu253Val	AACATTTTTGCAATTGTTCAATCTGT	
22	revHRPT2Leu253Val	TTTTACAGATTGAACAATTGCAAAA	
23	forHRPT2EcoRI	ATTAATTAGAATTCATGGCGGACGTGCTTA	pcDNA3-PFMR292K
24	revHRPT2XhoI	ATTAATTACTCGAGTCAGAATCTCAAGTGC	
25	forHRPT2Arg292Lys	CCCAGCTGCCTATAACAAATACGATCAGG	

26	revHRPT2Arg292Lys	CCTGATCGTATTTGTTATAGGCAGCTGGG	
27	forHRPT2EcoRI	ATTAATTAGAATTCATGGCGGACGTGCTTA	pcDNA3-PFMD379N
28	revHRPT2XhoI	ATTAATTACTCGAGTCAGAATCTCAAGTGC	
29	forHRPT2Asp379Asn	CCATGCTTAATGCAAAAAACCTTCTACAGGACC	
30	revHRPT2Asp379Asn	CAGGTCCTGTAGAAGGTTTTTTGCATTAAGCATGG	
31	forSki8EcoRI	ATTAATTAGAATTCATGACCAACCAGTACG	pcDNA3-Ski81-450* (EcoRI/XhoI)
32	revSki8450XhoI	ATTAATTACTCGAGTCAGAATTTTCCTCTAGTGT	
33	forSki8451EcoRI	ATTAATTAGAATTCATGATTCTTAGTATTGCATAT	pcDNA3-Ski8451-918* (EcoRI/XhoI)
34	revSki8XhoI	ATTAATTACTCGAGTTAAATTGGACAATCA	
35	forLeo1KpnI	ATTAATTAGGTACCATGGCGGATATGGAGGAT	pcDNA3-Leo11-1002* (XhoI/KpnI)
36	revLeo11002XhoI	ATTAATTACTCGAGTCAAGTAGGTGGTTTGTCTTC	
37	forLeo1003KpnI	ATTAATTAGGTACCATGCCAGGACAGCCTGTTGAT	pcDNA3-Leo11003-2004* (XhoI/KpnI)
38	revLeo1XhoI	ATTAATTACTCGAGTCAATCATCATCTTCTTC	
39	forPaf1EcoRI	ATTAATTAGAATTCATGGCGCCCACCATCCAG	pcDNA3-Paf11-798* (EcoRI/XhoI)
40	revPaf1798XhoI	ATTAATTACTCGAGTCACTCTTCTTACAGGCAGG	
41	forPaf1796EcoRI	ATTAATTAGAATTCATGGAGACGTTGAAGAAA	pcDNA3-Paf1-796-1608* (EcoRI/XhoI)
42	revPaf1XhoI	ATTAATTACTCGAGTCAGTCACTGTCACT	

4.7.3 Oligonucleotides for qRT-PCR

Number	Name	Target	Sequence
1	FKqPCR1h18Sfor	GTAACCCGTTGAACCCCATT	18S (mm, hs)
2	FKqPCR2h18Srev	CCATCCAATCGGTAGTAGCG	
3	HRPT2hfor19	GTCCTGCGACAGTACAACATC	HRPT2 (mm, hs)
4	HRPT2hrev157	CTCTGGGTTGGCCTTCCTTT	
5	P300forhSki	GTCCATAGATGCAGGACCTGT	Ski8
6	P498revhSki8	TCCACTGGCTAGGTATTTCCC	
7	P1261forhLeo1	AGATGGAGGATACGCCGAGAT	Leo1
8	P1478revhLeo1	GGTCTGAAGGTGAGTTTCGTTT	
9	P12forhCtr9	CTCCATCGAGATTCCCCTCC	Ctr9
10	P215revhCtr9	TTGCCATCTATACGTGCTGCT	
11	P49forhPaf1	CCCAATTCCCACCGGACTC	Paf1
12	P182revhPaf1	TACTGGACGATCCTGTTCTGG	
13	formusccnd1	GCGTACCCTGACACCAATCTC	Cyclin D1
14	revmusccnd1	CTCCTCTTCGCACTTCTGCTC	

15	formusIGF1	CTGGACCAGAGACCCTTTGC	IGF1
16	revmusIGF1	GGACGGGGACTTCTGAGTCTT	
17	formusIGF2	GTGCTGCATCGCTGCTTAC	IGF2
18	revmusIGF2	ACGTCCCTCTCGGACTTGG	
19	formusIGFBP4	AGAAGCCCCTGCGTACATTG	IGFBP1
20	revmusIGFBP4	TGTCCCCACGATCTTCATCTT	
21	formusHMGA1	GGTCGGGAGTCAGAAAGAGC	HMGA1
22	revmusHMGA1	ATTCTTGCTTCCCTTTGGTCG	
23	formusmyc	ATGCCCCTCAACGTGAACTTC	c-Myc
24	revmusmyc	CGCAACATAGGATGGAGAGCA	
25	musGAPDHfor	AGGTCGGTGTGAACGGATTTG	GAPDH
26	musGAPDHrev	TGTAGACCATGTAGTTGAGGTCA	

4.7.4 Oligonucleotides for antisense experiments

Name	Target	Application	Sequence	Supplier
PFM-1	HS HRPT2	Stable cell lines	TGCTGTTGACAGTGAGCGCCCAGTTGATATAT TTGCTAAATAGTGAAGCCACAGATGTATTTAG CAAATATATCAACTGGTTGCCTACTGCCTCGG A	Open Biosystems
PFM-2	HS and MM HRPT2	Stable and inducible cell lines	TGCTGTTGACAGTGAGCGCGGTTAAATTAGCA TTACTTAATAGTGAAGCCACAGATGTATTAAGT AATGCTAATTTAACCATGCCTACTGCCTCGGA	Open Biosystems
PFM-3	HS and MM HRPT2	Stable and inducible cell lines	TGCTGTTGACAGTGAGCGACCTTCTAGTCTGT AATGGAAATAGTGAAGCCACAGATGTATTTCC ATTACAGACTAGAAGGCTGCCTACTGCCTCGG A	Open Biosystems
Leo1-1	HS Leo1	Stable cell lines	TGCTGTTGACAGTGAGCGCGCAAAGAAACTTA CCAGTGATTAGTGAAGCCACAGATGTAATCAC TGGTAAGTTTCTTTGCTTGCCTACTGCCTCGG A	Open Biosystems
Ctr9-1	HS Ctr9	Stable cell lines	TGCTGTTGACAGTGAGCGCGAGGAGATGAAGTTA TCAGTATTTAGTGAAGCCACAGATGTAAATAC TGATAACTTCATCTCCCTGCCTACTGCCTCGG A	Open Biosystems
Ctr9-2	HS, MM and RN Ctr9	Stable cell lines	TGCTGTTGACAGTGAGCGCGCTACCTCTGTCC TGAAAGATTAGTGAAGCCACAGATGTAATCTT TCAGGACAGAGGTAGCTTGCCTACTGCCTCG GA	Open Biosystems
Ctr9-3	HS Ctr9	Stable cell lines	TGCTGTTGACAGTGAGCGAGCCTTGGTCCTG CAAAGATTATAGTGAAGCCACAGATGTATAAT CTTTGCAGGACCAAGGCCTGCCTACTGCCTC GGA	Open Biosystems
Ski8	HS Ski8	Stable cell lines	TGCTGTTGACAGTGAGCGCGCCATAGATGGA ATCATCAATTAGTGAAGCCACAGATGTAATTG ATGATTCCATCTATGGCTTGCCTACTGCCTCG GA	Open Biosystems
Non-silencing siRNA	Non-silencing	Transient transfections	ACGUGACACGUUCGGAGAAdTdT	QIAGEN
PFM-368	HS PFM	Transient transfections	CAUCUGCAGCUCGUUUGACdTdT	QIAGEN

4.7.5 Oligonucleotides for genotyping

Number	Name	Symbol in Results section	Sequence
1	1998	I	GGTTCAGGGCCCAAAACCTTATTAA
2	2000	II	AGGATGAGGTTCTTGCACTGGCAAG
3	2001	III	GTATTCCAACTGGCTTCCAAGC
4	2002	IV	AGTTTGTCTTCTATGGATAATCCTT

4.8 Plasmids

*numbers represent bp number

Number	Name	Source	Cloning strategy
1	pcDNA3		-
3	MSCV TMP	Ross Dickens (Hannon lab)	-
4	TMP-PFM-2	cloned by FK	EcoRI/XhoI
5	TMP-PFM-3	cloned by FK	EcoRI/XhoI
6	TMP-Leo1	cloned by FK	EcoRI/XhoI
7	TMP-Ctr9	cloned by FK	EcoRI/XhoI
8	TMP-Ski8	cloned by FK	EcoRI/XhoI
9	TMP-Paf1	cloned by FK	EcoRI/XhoI
10	MSCV LMP	Hannon lab	
11	LMP-NS	cloned by FK	EcoRI/XhoI
12	LMP-PFM-1	cloned by FK	EcoRI/XhoI
13	LMP-PFM-3	cloned by FK	EcoRI/XhoI
14	LMP-Leo1-1	cloned by FK	EcoRI/XhoI
15	LMP-Ctr9-1	cloned by FK	EcoRI/XhoI
16	LMP-Ctr9-2	cloned by FK	EcoRI/XhoI
17	LMP-Ski8	cloned by FK	EcoRI/XhoI
18	LMP-Paf1	cloned by FK	EcoRI/XhoI
19	pMal-c2	New England Biolaboratories	
20	pAcGHLT-A	BD Biosciences, modified by Christiane Wirbelauer, Krek lab	
21	pAcGHLT-A-Paf1	cloned by FK	SacI/KpnI
22	pAcGHLT-A-Leo1	cloned by FK	SacI/KpnI
23	pCMV-XL5-Ctr9	Reinberg lab	
24	pcDNA3-Ctr91-1749*	cloned by FK	XhoI/KpnI
28	pcDNA3-Ctr911749-3522*	cloned by FK	XhoI/KpnI
29	pGEX-4T1-PFM1-270 (PFM-NT)	Cloned by Armelle Yart, Krek lab	
30	pGEX-4T1-PFM270-531 (PFM-CT)	Cloned by Armelle Yart, Krek lab	
31	pcDNA3-HA-PFM	cloned by AY, Krek lab	
32	pcDNA3-PFM	cloned by AY, Krek lab	
33	pcDNA3-PFM2-222	cloned by AY, Krek lab	
34	pcDNA3-PFML253V	cloned by FK	PCR cloning
35	pcDNA3-PFM2-270	cloned by AY, Krek lab	
36	pcDNA3-PFM271-	cloned by AY, Krek lab	

		531		
37		pcDNA3-PFM222-263	cloned by FK	PCR cloning
38		pcDNA3-PFM222-271	cloned by FK	PCR cloning
39		pcDNA3-PFM371-531	cloned by FK	PCR cloning
40		pcDNA3-PFMR292K	cloned by FK	PCR cloning
41		pcDNA3-PFMK34Q	cloned by AY, Krek lab	
42		pcDNA3-PFML64P	cloned by AY, Krek lab	
43		pcDNA3-PFMD379N	cloned by FK	PCR cloning
44		pcDNA3-Ski8	cloned by FK	EcoRI/XhoI
45		pcDNA3-Ski81-450	cloned by FK	EcoRI/XhoI
46		pcDNA3-Ski8451-918*	cloned by FK	EcoRI/XhoI
47		pcDNA3-Leo1	Reinberg lab	
48		pcDNA3-flag-Leo1	Reinberg lab	
49		pcDNA3-Leo11-1002*	cloned by FK	XhoI/KpnI
50		pcDNA3-Leo11003-2004*	cloned by FK	XhoI/KpnI
51		pcDNA3-Paf1	AY, Krek lab	
52		pcDNA3-Paf11-798*	cloned by FK	EcoRI/XhoI
53		pcDNA3-Paf1-796-1608*	cloned by FK	EcoRI/XhoI
54		pcDNA3-URI	provided by Nabil Djouder, Krek lab	
55		psPAX2	Trono lab	
56		pMD2.G	Trono lab	
57		pBob-CAGGS-iCre-SD	Ian	
58		pSPORT-NEIL1		
56		pcDNA3-HIRA		
57		pcDNA3-MDM2	cloned by FK	
58		pSM2-shGFP		

4.9 Bacterial strains

All plasmids except for those with a pSM2 backbone were grown in the *E.coli* strain DH4α. Bacteria were cultured over night at 37°C in LB medium (liquid culture, shaken at 200rpm on a shaker for bacterial cultures) or on LB-Agar plates (solid cultures) in the presence of the respective antibiotics (Ampicilin: 100µg/mL, Chloramphenicol: 100µg/mL, Kanamycin: 50µg/mL). pSM2 plasmids were cultured in *E.coli pir1* in 2xLB medium and in the presence of Chloramphenicol (100µg/mL, shRNA insert selection marker) and Kanamycin (50µg/mL, vector selection marker).

4.10 Mammalian Cell lines

Number	Name	Tissue source	Origin
1	HeLa (+LMP plasmids)	human, Black, cervix, carcinoma, epitheloid	Helenius lab, puromycine for selection of stable knock downs: 2µg/mL,
2	NIH-3T3	mouse embryonic fibroblast cell line	NIH
3	LinX	NIH-3T3 murine fibroblast cell derived (mouse embryonic fibroblast)	NIH
4	Phoenix	NIH-3T3 murine fibroblast cell derived (mouse embryonic fibroblast)	NIH
5	786-O (+LMP plasmids)		Krek lab , puromycine for selection of stable knock downs: 786-O: 2µg/mL,
6	786-O + VHL (long)		Krek lab , 786-O +VHL: 3µg/mL neomycin selection of 786-O + VHL: 0,5µg/mL (1:100)
7	RCC-4 (+LMP plasmids)		
8	RCC-4 + VHL (long)		neomycin selection of 786-O + VHL: 0,5µg/mL (1:100);
9	RPE-1 (+LMP plasmids)	Retinal cell line	

| 10 | U2OS + rtTA (+TMP plasmids) | human osteosarcoma | neomycin selection of U2OS + rtTA: 0,5µg/mL (1:100); puromycin selection: 1µg/mL |
| 11 | PFM$^{fl/fl}$ MEFs | Mouse embryonic fibroblasts | 1,4µL β-mercaptoethanol was added to 100mL of normal growth medium |

4.11 Insect Cell lines

Sf9 cells (derived from ovarian tissue of *Spodoptera frugiperda*) were cultured in Grace's Insect Medium supplemented with Fetal Calf Serum.

4.12 Viruses

Number	Name of plasmid	Application
	Baculovirus	
1	pAcGHLT-A-GST	Production of GST in Sf9 cells
2	pAcGHLT-A-GST-URI	Production of GST-URI in Sf9 cells
3	pAcGHLT-A-GST-Leo1	Production of GST-Leo1 in Sf9 cells
4	pAcGHLT-A-GST-Ski8	Production of GST-Ski8 in Sf9 cells
5	pAcGHLT-A-GST-Ctr9	Production of GST-Ctr9 in Sf9 cells
6	pAcGHLT-A-GST-Paf1	Production of GST-Paf1 in Sf9 cells
7	pAcGHLT-A-GST-Parafibromin	Production of GST-Parafibromin in Sf9 cells
	Murine Embryonic Stem Cell Virus	
8	pSM2-shRNA-NS	Control for knock down experiments
9	pSM2-shRNA-Leo1	Stable knock down of Leo1 in human cancer cell lines
10	pSM2-shRNA-Ski8	Stable knock down of Ski8 in human cancer cell lines
11	pSM2-shRNA-Ctr9-1	Stable knock down of Ctr9 in human cancer cell lines
12	pSM2-shRNA-Ctr9-2	Stable knock down of Ctr9 in human cancer cell lines
13	pSM2-shRNA-Ctr9-3	Stable knock down of Ctr9 in human cancer cell lines
14	pSM2-shRNA-Paf1	Stable knock down of Paf1 in human cancer cell lines
15	pSM2-shRNA-Parafibromin-1	Stable knock down of Parafibromin in human cancer cell lines

16	pSM2-shRNA-Parafibromin-2	Stable knock down of Parafibromin in human cancer cell lines
17	pSM2-shRNA-Parafibromin-3	Stable knock down of Parafibromin in human cancer cell lines
18	LMP-shRNA-NS	Control for knock down experiments
19	LMP-shRNA-Leo1	Stable knock down of Leo1 in human cancer cell lines
20	LMP-shRNA-Ski8	Stable knock down of Ski8 in human cancer cell lines
21	LMP-shRNA-Ctr9-1	Stable knock down of Ctr9 in human cancer cell lines
22	LMP-shRNA-Ctr9-2	Stable knock down of Ctr9 in human cancer cell lines
23	LMP-shRNA-Ctr9-3	Stable knock down of Ctr9 in human cancer cell lines
24	LMP-shRNA-Paf1	Stable knock down of Paf1 in human cancer cell lines
25	LMP-shRNA-Parafibromin-1	Stable knock down of Parafibromin in human cancer cell lines
26	LMP-shRNA-Parafibromin-2	Stable knock down of Parafibromin in human cancer cell lines
27	LMP-shRNA-Parafibromin-3	Stable knock down of Parafibromin in human cancer cell lines
28	TMP-shRNA-Parafibromin-1	Inducible knock down of Parafibromin in human cancer cell lines
29	TMP-shRNA-Parafibromin-2	Inducible knock down of Parafibromin in human cancer cell lines
30	TMP-shRNA-Parafibromin-3	Inducible knock down of Parafibromin in human cancer cell lines
	Adenovirus	
31	pCre	Excision of $PFM^{fl/fl}$ in MEFs
	Lentivirus	
32	LVTHM	Control for knock down experiments
33	LVTHM-sh695	Stable knock down of Parafibromin in human cancer cell lines
34	LVTHM-sh695-HA-PFM-R222X	Stable knock down of Parafibromin and reconstitution with Parafibromin-R222X in human cancer cell lines

Part II: Methods in Molecular Biology, Proteinbiochemistry, Cell Biology

4.13 Isolation of DNA

4.13.1 Isolation of plasmid DNA from bacterial cultures (Mini, Midi, Maxi)

Bacteria clones were cultured in 2mL (Minipreps), 50mL (Midipreps) or 100mL (Maxipreps) over night at 37°C in LB medium (liquid culture, shaken at 200rpm on a shaker for bacterial cultures) in the presence of the respective antibiotics (ampicilin: 100µg/mL, chloramphenicol: 100µg/mL, kanamycin: 50µg/mL). Plasmids from Midi and Maxi cultures were purified using „Nucleobond plasmid purification procedure" (MACHERY-NAGEL). For that, bacterial clones were cultured ON and centrifuged at 6000xg for 15min at 4°C. The bacterial cells were lysed in 4mL (12mL for Maxi) buffer S1 + RNase A. 4mL (12mL for Maxi) of Buffer S2 was added in a second step, the tube inverted 6-8 times and incubated at RT for 2-3min. To lyse the cells, 4mL (12mL for Maxi) of pre-cooled buffer S3 was added, the lysate inverted and incubated for 5min on ice. In the meantime, the Nucleobond folded filter was placed in a funnel on top of the Nucleobond column. The filter was then prewetted and the column equilibrated with 5mL (10mL for Maxi) of buffer N2 before the bacterial lysate was poured into the filter and through the column. The column was washed with 10mL (32mL for Maxi) of buffer N3 and the plasmid eluted with 5mL (15mL) of buffer N5. The eluted plasmid DNA was then precipitated by addition of 3.5mL (11mL for Maxi) of isopropanol. The precipiate was then centrifuged for 30min at 15000xg at 4°C, washed in 2mL (5mL) of 70% Ethanol and the suspension transfered into Eppendorf tubes. In a last step, the precipitate was centrifuged the supernatant carefully removed and the pellet dried at RT for 5-10min (10-20min for Maxi) before the purified plasmid DNA was dissolved in H_2O and the concentration determined by UV photospectroscopy (Ultraspec Pro, Amersham Biosciences).

Plasmids from Miniprep cultures were purified using QIAprep Spin Miniprep Kit" using a microcentrifuge (Qiagen) according to the manufacturers instructions. For that the bacterial pellet was resuspended in 250µL of Buffer P1 (that contained RNase A). Cells were lysed by adding 250µL of buffer P2 and inverting the tube gently 4-6 times. After 2-3min incubation at RT, 350µL of Buffer N3 was added and the tube inverted 4-6 times to precipitate the genomic DNA and proteins. The tube was then centrifuged for 10min at 13000rpm in a table-top microcentrifuge for 10min and the resulting supernatants decanted into a QIAprep spin column. The DNA was bound to the column through a short centrifugation step (11000rpm in a table-top microcentrifuge at RT for 1min) and the column washed with 750µL of Buffer PE. An additional short centrifugation step (11000rpm in a table-top microcentrifuge at RT for 1min) removed all residual wash buffer, the DNA was eluted in 50µL of H_2O and the concentration determined by UV photospectroscopy (Ultraspec Pro, Amersham Biosciences).

4.13.2 Isolation of genomic DNA for genotyping of MEFs

20µL of MEF cell pellet was lysed in 75µL of hot Shot Lysis Buffer (25mM NaOH, 0.2mM EDTA-NaOH, pH 12) for 15min at 100°C, before the WCE were neutralized with Hot Shot Neutralization Buffer (40mM Tris, pH 5) for 2min on ice.

4.13.3 Isolation of DNA from Agarose gels using the QIAEX II Agarose Gel Extraction Protocol

DNA was amplified via PCR and separated on a 1% agarose gel, before bands were analysed under UV light and excised with a raiser blade. The excised slice was weighted 300µL of buffer QX1 and 200µL of H_2O was added per 100mg gel. Then, 30µL of well-mixed QIAEX II, which consists of beats, was added. The mix was then incubated at 50°C for 10min to solubilize the gel and bind the DNA to the beats. The mix was vortexed every two minutes to keep the QIAEX beats in solution. In a next step, 10µL of 3M $Na^+CH_2COO^-$, pH 5.0 (NaOH to titrate pH), and the mix incubated for 5min. Samples were centrifuged for 30s (Eppendorf table centrifuge) and the supernatant carefully removed with a pipette. The following washing steps consisted of adding the buffer, vortexing the sample, recovering the pellet by centrifuging it for

30s and removing the supernatant carefully with a pipette. In the first washing step, 500µL of Buffer QXI was used, in the second and third step each time 700µL Buffer PE. The pellet was then dried at 50°C for approximately 10min until it became white and the DNA eluted from the beats by resuspending them in 20µL of H_2O. In a last step, samples were centrifuged for 30s and the supernatant containing the DNA removed with a pipette.

4.14 Isolation of RNA

RNA isolation was performed according to the total RNA Isolation protocol from Macherey-Nagel. For that $1\text{-}5*10^6$ cells were harvested and lysed in 350µL of RA1 buffer supplemented with 3.5µL of β-mercaptoethanol before they were filtered through NucleoSpin® Filter Units by centrifugation at 11000xg for 1min in a microcentrifuge. 350µL of 70% ethanol (DEPC-treated dH_2O was used for dilution: 1mL of DEPC were added to 1L of dH_2O, the solution vigorously shaken and incubated at RT ON in a fume hood before it was autoclaved) was added to the homogenized lysate, which was then added into a NucleoSpin® RNAII column and centrifuged for 30s at 8000xg in a microcentrifuge. The silica membrane was desalted by adding 350µL of membrane desalting buffer and centrifuging for 1min at 11000xg. In a next step, bound DNA was removed by incubating 95µL of DNase reaction buffer (solution of 10µL of reconstituted DNase I and of 90µL of DNase reaction buffer) for 15min at RT on the column. After that, the column was washed with 200µL of RA2, with 600µL of RA3 (both times centrifuged at 8000xg for 30s) and with 250µL of RA3 and the membrane dried by centrifugion at 11000xg for 2min. The RNA was finally eluted by pipetting 60µL of DEPC-treated dH_2O onto the membrane and centrifugation at 11000xg for 1min.

4.15 Quantification of Nucleic Acids

The concentration of DNA and RNA was measured with a Ultraspec Pro, Amersham Biosciences at 260nm and 280nm. The concentrations were calculated using the following formula:

$$(DNA \text{ or } RNA)\left[\frac{\mu g}{\mu L}\right] = k \cdot A_{260} \cdot D$$

with: k : constant factor (for dsDNA k = 50µg/µL and for ssRNA k = 40µg/µL)
A_{260} : extinction at 260nm
D : dilution factor

The cleanness of the DNA and RNA was determined by calculating the ratio A_{260}/A_{280}. Thereby, a solution with a ratio A_{260}/A_{280} of >1.8 was considered as a pure solution, values below 1.8 indicated the presence of proteins.

4.16 Restriction enzyme digestions

All restriction enzymes were purchased from Roche or New England Biolaboratories and all digestions were performed according to the manufacturers protocols. For that, DNA was digested in a solution of 10% of RE Buffer, 2.5% of (each) RE, 1% BSA (if recommended).

Double digestions were except for very few cases carried out simultaneously.

4.17. Ligation of DNA fragments

DNA fragments were ligated using the Rapid Ligation kit from Roche. For that 1µL of RE-digested plasmid was added to 7µL of RE-digested plasmid (molar ratio of plasmid vs insert of approximately 1:5) and 2µL of 1xDNA dilution buffer. The solution was mixed well before 10µL of Ligase buffer and 1µL of T4 DNA ligase were added. After 5min incubation at RT, the ligated DNA was transformed into bacteria.

4.17.1 Liquid Culture

Bacteria were grown in LB medium containing the respective antibiotic resistance marker at 200rpm at 37°C. For long term storage, 1mL of bacterial suspension added to 500µL of 60% sterile glycerole was stored at -80°C. To re-culture bacteria a few µL of the suspension were either pipetted or scraped off and added into the prepared sterile LB medium.

4.17.2 Solid Culture

For selection of bacteria clones, 20-40µL of bacteria were dispersed on a culture dish with LB-Agar and the respective antibiotics and incubated ON at 37°C.

4.17.3 Transformation of bacteria

In a first step, competent *E. coli* (DH5α) were thawed on ice and mixed with the plasmid. After an incubation time of 20min on ice, the bacteria were heat-shocked at 42°C for 90s and transferred back on ice for 2min. 20-50µL of the cell suspension was then pipetted onto a LB-Amp culture dish and dispersed. The plate was then incubated overnight at 37°C, before colonies were picked and cultured overnight in 1mL of LB-media supplemented with Ampicillin in snap caps.

4.18 Preparation of competent Bacteria *E. coli* (DH5α)

Ten large colonies of freshly grown *E. coli* (DH5α) were cultured ON at 26°C in 400mL of sterilized SOB-NaOH medium pH 7.0 (20g/L of Bacto tryptone, 5g/L of Bacto yeast extract, 0.5g/L of NaCl, 2.5mM KCl, 10mM $MgCl_2$). At an OD_{600} of 0.45 the culture was dsplit into eight sterile 50mL Falcon tubes and placed on ice for 10min before they were centrifuged for 15min at 2500xg. The cell pellets were then pooled by carefully resuspending them in 128mL of filter sterilized HTB pH 6.7 (10mM HEPES-HCl, 15mM $CaCl_2$, 250mM KCl, 55mM $MnCl_2$). In the last step, 2.4mL of sterile DMSO was slowly added whle gently swirling the suspension and the competent bacteria stored at -80°C in 200µL aliquots.

4.19 Agarose Gel electrophoresis

All ethidium bromide stained gels were visualized under UV light and photographed on uvidoc system (Witec AG) black and white prints.

DNA was separated on 1% (w/v) Agarose gels. For this, 1% (w/v) Agarose was dissolved in 1x Tris-Borate-EDTA-buffer (1L of 10xTBE-buffer: 108g Tris-HCl, 55g boric acid, 40mL of 0.5M Na_2EDTA, pH 8.0, titrated with NaOH) by boiling it up in the microwave. 2-5µL of the DNA-intercalating agent Ethidium Bromide was added and the Agarose solution poured into the gel chambers. The DNA samples, diluted in 10% (v/v) of 10x gel loading buffer were pipetted into the wells of the gel. Agarose Gels were then run in 1x TBE-Buffer at 100V.

4.20 Purification of proteins

4.20.1 Affinity purification using the GST-tag

2x100mL of the *E.coli* clone suspension was cultured ON at 37°C in the presence of ampicilin. On the next morning, 900mL of LB-Amp medium was added to each culture and the cultures incubated for 1h at 37°C. To induce production of the GST fusion protein, 1mL of 0.1M stock IPTG was added and the cultures grown for 3h, before the cultures were transferred into 1/2L plastic centrifuge bottles and centrifuged for 5min at 4000xg. The supernatant was discarded and the bacteria pellets frozen at -20°C ON. On the next morning, the pellets were resuspended in 50mL of freshly prepared NETN buffer (20mM Tris-HCl pH=7.5, 1M NaCl, 1mM EDTA, 0.05% Nonidet P40, 1mM PMSF, 0.5mM DTT). The suspensions were pooled to two 100mL suspensions and sonicated four times for 10s at full power on a sonicator on ice. Each lysate was divided into four high-speed centrifugation tubes and spun at 17000xg for 10min at 4°C. For purification of the GST fusion proteins, the supernatants were transferred into four 50mL Falcon tubes and incubated with 800µL of glutathione sepharose beads (400µL per culture) for 2h at 4°C. Afterwards, the beads were spun down for 1min at 1500xg, resuspended in 1mL of NETN buffer and transferred to

Eppendorf tubes. Beads were incubate for 5min at 4°C on a head-over-tail rotator and washed three times with 1mL of NETN buffer and the forth time with 50mM Tris-HCl at pH=7.5 (same centrifugation conditions). After removal of the supernatant, the fusion protein was eluted with 250µL, 150µL and 150µL of 15mM reduced Glutathione in 50mM NaCl and 50mM Tris-HCl ph=8.1. Finally, the protein concentration was determined in a Bradford assay. the purified protein visualized on a PAA gel and the proteins stored in 35% glycerole at -80°C.

For the *in vitro* binding assay, GST fusion proteins were not produced in *E. coli*, but in Sf9 cells. For that, Sf9 cells were infected with Baculovirus harbouring an insert that encoded the desired GST fusion protein. After 2d, Sf9 cells were harvested, spun down at 2000xg and lysed in 500µL of TNN buffer (50mM Tris-HCl pH=7.5, 250mM NaCl, 5mM EDTA, 0.5% NP-40, 50mM NaF, 0.5mM DTT, 1µg/mL Aprotinin, 1mM PMSF) on a head-over-tail rotator for 20min at 4°C. After centrifugation for 15min at 13000rpm at 4°C on a tabletop microcentrifuge, the supernatant was added to 200µL of glutathione sepharose beads. Washing steps were performed as described above (proteins were not eluted but used immobilized on the beads).

4.20.2 Affinity purification using the MBP-tag

Bacteria were cultured, induced, harvested and lysed as described for the purification of GST fusion proteins. Instead of glutathione sepharose beads, 500µL of amylose beads were incubated with the lysate for 2h at 4°C. Beads were spun down for 1min at 1500xg and washed four times in 5mL of washing buffer (20mM Tris-HCl pH=7.5, 0.2M NaCl, 1mM EDTA, 0.5mM DTT). The fusion proteins were eluted through addition of 350µL of Laemmli Buffer and incubation at 100°C for 5min. The concentration of purified protein was measured by Bradford assay and purity analyzed by PAGE and WB.

4.21 Purification of polyclonal antibodies against parafibromin

4.21.1 Preparation of the affitnity column for antibody purification

MBP-taged parafibromin was produced in *E.coli* and purified as described. To prepare the affinity column, 4mL of amylose resin was added to the purified MBP-PFM and incubated for 4h at 4°C on a shaker. The MBP-PFM-resin was centrifuged für 2min at 1000rpm, the supernatant discarded and the beads washed twice with 10mL of 0.2M Na-Borate pH 9.0 (3mL of 0.2M boric acid pH 4.0 and 27mL of 0.05M Borax pH 10, titrated with NaOH) for 5min at 4°C. The resin was then centrifugated for 5min at 1000rpm and washed with 10mL of Na-Borate. After centrifugation (same conditions), the fusion protein was coupled by incubating the beads for 1h at RT in 10mL of Na-Borate supplemented with 103.6mg of DMP. After coupling, the beads were washed with 10mL of 0.2M ethanolamine-HCl pH 8.0 before they were incubated in ethanolamine for 2h at RT. Subsequently, the beads were washed twice with 10mL of cold PBS and stored in PBS supplemented with 0.05% NaN_3.

4.21.2 Purification and dialysis of polyclonal antibodies

The MBP-PFM column was washed with 10mL of PBST (PBS supplemented with 0.2% Tween20), then with 10mL of 0.2M Glycine-HCl pH2.2, followed by washing with 10mL of freshly prepared 100mM Triethanolamine-HCl pH 11.5 and finally again with 10mL of PBST. Meanwhile, 3mL of serum were diluted in 7mL of PBST and then passed through the column, which was then washed approximately four times with PBST at 4°C until the OD_{280} of the flowthrough reached 0.01. The purified antibodies were finally eluted with 8-10mL of Glycine-HCl pH 2.2. To neutralize the aliquots 250µL L of 1M K_2HPO_4 were added to each 750µL of eluate. For storage, the column was washed again with PBS and stored at 4°C in PBS supplemented with 0.05% NaN_3. The OD of the eluates was meassured with a Ultraspec Pro, Amersham Biosciences at 280nm and the three to four fractions with the highest OD pooled, dialysed against PBS + 30% glycerole ON at 4°C using a 6-8kD membrane (Spectrumlabs). Concentrated antibodies were tested for functionality and stored at -80°C.

4.22 DNA sequencing

DNA was sequenced by Microsynth under standard conditions.

4.23 PCR

4.23.1 PCR

PCR was carried out according to the manufacturers protocols. Taq DNA Polymerase (Invitrogen) was used for standard PCR like genotyping and Pwo DNA Polymerase (Roche) or Pfu DNA Polymerase (Catalysis) were used in all cloning experiments (the volume of each reaction was 25µL, final primer conc. was 5µM, final dNTP conc. was 0.2µM, all reactions contained specific PCR reaction buffer, 0.25µL of DMSO was added to Pfu).

4.23.2 Reverse transcriptase PCR

Reverse transcriptase PCR were done using either the „ Superscript™ First Strand Synthesis System for RT-PCR" (Invitrogen) or the „Ready-to-Go You-Prime First-Strand-Beads" from (GE Healthcare) according to manufacturers description.

Superscript™ First-Strand Synthesis System:

1μL of 10mM dNTP mix and 1μL of 0.5μg/μL oligo(dT)$_{12-18}$ was added to 8μL DNAse I treated mRNA. The RNA was then denatured at 65°C for 5min and incubated at 4°C for 1min. In a next step, 2μL of 10x Reverse Transcriptase (RT) buffer, 4μL of 25mM MgCl$_2$, 2μL of 0.1 M DTT and 1μL of RNaseOUT™ Recombinant RNase Inhibitor were added to each sample. The annealing step was carried out at 42°C for 2min, before 50u ($\hat{=}$1μL) of SuperScript™ II RT was mixed into each tube. The subsequent cDNA synthesis was performed at 42°C for 50min, the reactions terminated at 70°C for 15min and the samples chilled on ice. The contents of each tube was briefly centrifuged to the bottom of each tube and the remaining RNA digested by adding 1μL of RNase H (Invitrogen, 2u/μL Cat. #18021-071) for 20min at 37°C.

Alternatively, cDNA-synthesis was carried out using „Ready-To-Go You-Prime First-Strand Beads" (GE Healthcare) according to the manufacturer's instructions. For that, 100ng to 3μg of total RNA in a volume of 29μL were heated at 65°C for 10min, then chilled on ice for 2min. RNA was then added to the beads and 4μL of random hexamers before the mix was incubated for 1min at RT.The tube was vortexed and briefly centrifuged on a table-top microcentrifuge, and incubated at 37°C for 1h. 2-5μL of this first-strand reaction was used in downstream QPCR experiments.

4.23.3 Quantitative PCR

QPCRs were performed with the Lightcycler system from Roche. Optical plates and clear adhesive seal was supplied by Applied Biosystems. Each reaction had a total volume of 20µL (10µL of SYBR Green PCR master mix, 250nM of each primer). The C_T-values were determined using the software and the fold of expression change for each of the genes were calculated according to the following formula:

$$fold\ change = 2^{\Delta C_T}$$

The values for each gene were normilized by dividing their fold change by the fold change of the housekeeping gene 18S rRNA.

4.24 Cell Culture

4.24.1 Cell culture of the immortalized insect cell Sf9

Sf9 cells were grown at 28°C until confluency and splitted 1:6. For that, cells were washed twice with sterile PBS and recovered with medium. Cells were then detached with one hit against the flask and the floating cells were finally dispersed on cell culture flasks continaing fresh medium.

For freezing, Sf9 cells were washed with PBS and detached as described above. Cells were then centrifuged for 10min at 1000xg, the pellet resuspended in freezing medium (30% fetal calf serum, 10% DMSO in Grace's Insect medium) and the cells kept at -80°C (transferred to liquid N_2 for longterm storage after 1-8 weeks). As DMSO is toxic to cells, it was worked rather quickly once the cells came in contact with the freezing solution. 1mL aliquots were then transferred into cryo vials and frozen down at -80C. Cells were stored at -80°C for periods of up to 3 weeks and were transferred into N_2 (l) (approximately -196°C) for longer storage periods.

Sf9 cells were gently thawed in a 37°C water bath, spun at 600xg for 3min and resuspended in fresh medium.

4.24.2 Generation and amplification of Baculovirus

$2*10^6$ Sf9 cells were seeded in a 6cm dish (50-70% density) at day 1. In a second step, 0.5µg of BaculoGold DNA was added to 2µg of recombinant baculovirus transfer vector containing the insert. The tube was mixed well by gentle vortexing and incubated at RT for 5min before 1mL of Transfection Buffer B was added. In a third step, the Sf9 cell medium was replaced by 1mL of Transfection Buffer A before the Transfection Buffer B/ DNA mixture was added to the cell in a dropwise manner (the plate was gently rocked after every 3-5 drops). The plate was incubated for 4h at 27°C before the transfection medium was replaced with 3mL of fresh medium. After 4-5 days, the cells were harvested and assayed for expression of the transgene by western blotting. The supernatant was filtered through a Nalgene 0.45µm PES membrane. To amplify the virus, a second 6cm dish of $2*10^6$ Sf9 cells was then infected with the filtered virus-containing supernatant. After 4-5 days cell were checked for signs of infection (floating cells). This amplification step was repeated once to twice until infection of Sf9 cells became visible. The virus-containing supernatant was stored at 4°C in the dark (storage for up to several months) and in small aliquots at -80°C (storage for years). For re-infection, 1mL of stored supernatant was added to an $80cm^2$ flask of Sf9 cells;

4.24.3 Cell culture mammalian cell lines (splitting, freezing, thawing)

Mammalian cell lines were grown in standard DMEM supplemented with 10% FCS and Glutamin at 37°C and 5% CO_2. To avoid overgrowth and spontaneous differentiation the immortalized cell lines were split every few days. For this, medium was removed and cells were washed twice with PBS. Trypsin was added to the cells and the cells were incubated at 37°C for 3min. Serum containing medium was added to inhibit Trypsin and the cell suspension was spun for 3min at 3000rpm. Subsequently, the supernatant was discarded and 2mL of media was added to the pelletized cells. In a next step, cells were dissociated by triturating them 3 to 4 times, redissolved and plated on a new dish.

For long-term storage, cells were washed twice with 1xPBS before and trypsinized at 37°C. Serum containing medium was added, cells were harvested and centrifuged for 3min at 2000xg. The supernatant was discarded and the cells were dissolved in cold freezing medium [10% (v/v) DMSO in serum-containing medium]. 1mL aliquots were then transferred into cryo vials and frozen down at -80C. Cells were stored at -80°C for periods of up to 3 weeks and were transferred into N_2 (l) (approximately -196°C) for longer storage periods.

For thawing, a cryo vial containing the frozen cells was placed in a 37°C dH_2O bath until contents were completely thawed. Approximately 1mL of appropriate medium was added and mixed into the cell suspension by repeatedly soaking the cell suspension up and releasing it into the vial again. Then, the suspension was centrifuged for 3min at 2000xg and the supernatant discarded. The cells were triturated three to four times to dissociate the cells and 2mL of media was added. The cells were then plated onto a dish and incubate at 37°C.

4.24.4 Preparation of primary mouse embryonic fibroblasts

Pfm$^{wt/fl}$ mice were crossed ON. After 14d, pregnant female mice were sacrificed using a CO_2 and wetted with Ethanol (to prevent subsequent contamination). Forelimbs and hidelimbs were fixed and the mouse cut open at the skin of the fur. Each embryo was isolated from the uterus and collected in 6cm dish with sterile cold PBS supplemented with 2%FCS on ice. Yolk bag, placenta, head and all organs were removed and the remaining embryos collected in a fresh 6cm dish with sterile cold PBS supplemented with 2%FCS on ice. After every embryo had been treated, they were transferred to a clean bench in the cell culture laboratory. For each embryo, 2mL of Trypsin was added into a 10cm petri dish and each embryo was chopped into tiny pieces. Once each embryo nhad become almost liquid, it was moved into the Trypsin and incubated at 37°C for 15min. In the last step, the embryonic cells were dispersed by pipetting several times up and down with a 1mL pipette, added into 10cm MEF medium (DMEM, 10%FCS, 1% Glutamin, 1% Pen/Strep, 200µM β-mercaptoethanol) and incubated at 37°C. After 3-4d, MEFs were confluent and cultured and frozen according to standard procedure.

4.24.5 Counting of mammalian and insect cells

Cell suspensions were 1:10 diluted in Trypan Blue and counted using a hemocytometer. For this, cells were pipetted onto the hemocytometer and counted in each quadrant of the grid. This step was repeated at least once and the numbers averaged. The cell number was calculated according to the following formula:.

$$n(cells) = \overline{x} \cdot D \cdot 10^4$$

with: n(cells) : number of cells
 $\overline{x}$: arithmetic mean in quadrant
 d : dilution factor

4.24.6 Retroviral transduction of mammalian cell lines and long-term storage of viruses

To produce retrovirus expressing cell lines, different mammalian cell lines were transfected with the respective constructs. Since the transfection methods used were dependend on the type of virus, each method is separately described in the following.

4.24.7 Calcium-Phosphate Transfection of 293T cells to produce Lentivirus and infection of target cell lines

On day 1, 2.5×10^5 293T cells were plated on a 6cm dish and incubated in the incubator in growth medium without antibiotics. On the evening of day 2, the cells were transfected. For that, sterilefiltered 2xHBS pH 6.90 stored at -20°C (25mL of 50mM Na-HEPES-HCl, pH 7.05, 10mM KCl, 280mM NaCl, 1.5 mM Na_2HPO_4 x $2H_2O$, 12 mM glucose) was slowly thawed at RT. For each dish 500µL of 2xHBS was aliquoted in sterile Eppendorf tubes. In separate tubes, 20µg of plasmid DNA, 15µg of psPAX2 and 6µm of pMD2 were added to 61µL of sterilefiltered 2M $CaCl_2$ solution (stored at -20°C). dH_2O was added to bring the DNA/ $CaCl_2$ solution to a final volume of 500µL. In a next step, the DNA/ $CaCl_2$ solution was added to the 2xHBS solution and the solution mixed. The transfection solution was then added drop by drop evenly to the cells. Avoiding to shake the dish, the cells were transferred to 37°C and incubated ON. On day 3, growth medium was exchanged and cell incubated for another 2-3d. On day 4-5, the supernatant was collected, separated from the cells by centrifugation (3min at 3000rpm) and filtered through 0.45µm filters. Infection of the target cell line was performed only with fresh supernatant.

4.24.8 Transfection of LinX cells to produce murine embyronic stem cell virus

On day 1, $3*10^6$ LinX cells were plated on a 10cm dish (30-40% density on day 2) and incubated ON in growth medium without antibiotics. The next day, 250µL of DMEM with 15µg of plasmid (encoding the hairpin) were added to 250µL of DMEM supplemented with 75µg of FUGENE. The solution was mixed and incubated at RT for 10min before it was added to 4.5mL of DMEM to yield the transfection medium. Subsequently, the old growth medium was removed and the cell incubated in transfection medium for 4-6h before 5mL of growth medium without antibiotics was added to the cells. On the third day 2, medium was exchanged and on day 4 the virus containing supernatant centrifuged and filtered through 0.45µm filters. The supernatant were stored at -80°C and 5mL of the supernatants were used to infect target cell lines.

4.24.9 Generation of cell lines, which inducibly or stably downregulate Paf1C components

MSCV containing supernatants were supplemented with 5µg/mL polybrene (polycation, which reduces charge repulsion between virus and cell membrane) and added to the target cell lines. 24h later, medium was exchanged and selection with 0.3-6µg/mL of puromycine (cell line dependent) started. The selection period typically lasted for 5-7d.

In the case of inducible expression of the shRNA, MSCV containing supernatants were added to U2OS cells expressing the reverse transcriptional transactivator (rtTA). Furthermore and in contrast to the generation of stable cell lines, clonal cell lines were generated. For that, clones that emerged during the puromycine selection were covered with cloning discs (SIGMA-Aldrich). After a couple of days, the discs were picked with forceps and transferred into 24-wells, were they were expanded, tested and eventually frozen for long-term-storage. To test for inducible expression of the sh RNA clones were cultured in 100ng/mL of doxycycline for 8d, harvested and the downregulation of the target genes analyzed by QPCR (RNA level) and by WB (protein level).

4.24.10 Production of Adenovirus expressing Cre-recombinase

The growth medium of a 80% confluent 80cm^2 flask of 293 cells was exchanged for infection medium (growth medium with 5% FCS instead of 10%) and purified Adeno-Cre virus added to the cells. After 3-5 days incubation, cells were flushed off by pipetting and centrifuged at 1200rpm for 5min. Except for 10mL, the complete supernant was then removed and the cell pellet resuspended. After four freeze-thaw cycles in N_2 (l) at in a 37°C water bath (supension was stirred during thawing) and cellular debris was separated from the supernatant by centrifugation for 15min at 4000rpm. The supernatant was then filtered through 0.45µm filters and used to re-infect a 80% confluent 75cm^2 flask of 293 cells to amplify the virus.

Adeno-Cre virus was purified using the Vivapure® AdenoPack™ 20 procedure (Sartorius) accordig to the manufacturers instructions. For that 1µL of Benzonase was added to each mL of virus containing supernatant, the solution mixed well and incubated at 37°C for 30min. The nuceic acid digested supernatant was then loaded onto a Vivaclear Maxi and spun for at 500xg until the whole volume had passed the membrane. The flow-through was collected and 1/9 volume of 10x loading buffer added under agitation. In a next step, an AdenoPACK 20 Maxi spin column was equilibrated with 5mL of 1x washing buffer (spun for 5min at 500rpm), the sample loaded and the column spun for 500xg until the sample had completely passed. Subsequently, the spin column was washed twice with 18mL of 1x washing buffer. Finally, 1mL elution buffer was pipetted onto the membrane, the column spun for 30s at 500rpm before the column was incubated at RT or 10min and centrifuged for 5min at 500rpm.

4.25 Isolation of proteins

Mammalian cells were harvested, spun down at 2000xg and lysed in 500µL of TNN buffer (50mM Tris-HCl pH=7.5, 250mM NaCl, 5mM EDTA, 0.5% NP-40, 50mM NaF, 0.5mM DTT, 1µg/mL Aprotinin, 1mM PMSF) on a head-over-tail rotator for 20min at 4°C. After lysis, cells were centrifuged for 15min at 13000rpm at 4°C on a table-top microcentrifuge and the supernatant used as the WCE.

4.26 Quantification of proteins

4.26.1 Bradford Assay

To quantify proteins, 5-10µL of protein solutions were added into 1.5mL of 1x Bradford solution (Biorad-Protein Assay 1:5 diluted in dH_2O). After 15-20min of incubation, the absorption at 595nm was determined using the Ultraspec Pro (Amersham Biosciences). The standard curve was calculated after parallel determination of absorption at 595nm of known masses of BSA (0µg, 5µg, 7.5µg, 10µg and 12.5µg) using the same assay.

4.26.2 Colloidal Coomassie Staining

Following electrophoresis, the PAG was placed into colloidal coomassie staining solution (13.51mL of 85% ortho-phosphoric acid, 100g of ammonium sulfate, 1g of Coomassie Brilliant Blue G250 and 200mL of methanol were diluted in dH_2O and brought to a volume of 1000mL) for 6-12h. The gel was then destained on a shaker at RT with several changes of dH_2O. Coomassie stained gels were digitalized using the Odyssey system (any wavelengths).

4.27 Production of polyclonal antibodies

Polyclonal antibodies against the N-terminal and C-terminal half of parafibromin were produced with the help of Bogdan Gerya and Felix Hauler and with Eurogentec S.A.. During this project, GST fusion proteins of the N-terminal and C-terminal half of parafibromin were produced in bacteria and purified as described. The protein concentration and the purity of the eluates were analyzed by the Bradford assay and Coomassie staining. At Eurogentec S.A., 100µg of each antigen, was injected per rabbit. One rabbit was sacrificed after six immunizations, all remaining rabbits were immunized for nine times. The serum was purified as described.

4.28 Denaturing (SDS) discontinous Polyacrylamide gelelectrophoresis (PAGE)

The protein concentration of WCE was quantified using the Bradford assay. 20-100µg of proteins were then pipetted to 3µL of Laemmli buffer (0.125M Trizma, 0.96M glycine, 0.5% SDS) and heated for 3min at 99°C. The glass-plate sandwich (containing a glass plate, an aluminium plate, two plastic spacer and a comb) was assembled and the 6-15% separating gel and on top of it the stacking gel casted. The WCE were loaded and the SDS- polyacrylamide gel electrophoresis system from

Hoefer used to separate the proteins at 120V on SDS PAGE running buffer (1g of SDS, 3.03g of Tris, 14.41g of glycin) at RT.

4.29 Western Blotting and Immunodetection of proteins

After PAGE, proteins were electrophoretically transfered to a 0.45µm nitrocellulose membrane (Schleicher & Schuell) in a tank. For that, the stacking gel was removed and the transfer tank (Anode - Whatman paper – in transfer buffer prewetted membrane - PAG - Whatmanpaper - Kathode) assembled and inserted into the blotting tank with transfer buffer (14.4g/L of glycine, 5.8g/L of Tris, 20% of methanol). The proteins were transferred at 600mA for 2-12h at 4°C.

After the transfer, the NC membrane was blocked in TBST supplemented with 5% nonfat dried milk (blotto) for 30min at RT on a shaker. Subsequently, the blotto was exchanged for in blotto diluted antibody and incubated for either 2h at RT or ON at 4°C on a shaker. After three washing steps with TBST for 10min each, the respective secondary antibody was diluted in TBST and added to the membrane for 1h. Three further washing steps of TBST for 10min each at RT removed excess antibodies and prepared the membrane fort he detection of specific protein bands.

The main method used for detection is described in the following:

4.29.1 Odyssey system

The wet membrane was placed on the scanner and scaned for fluorescent signals at the respective wavelength (680nm and 800nm). If a reblotting with another antibody was planned, it was ensured that the membrane remained wet. For long-term storage, the membrane was dried and kept at 4°c in the dark.

4.30 Fluorescent Activated Cell Sorting (FACS)

Cells were trypsinized and harvested by centrifugation, before they were resuspended in PBS. While vortexing, 1mL of -20°C cold 100% Ethanol was added dropwise and the cells incubated at -20°C in the dark ON. On the next day, cells were washed with 1mL of PBS (centrifugation step at 1400rpm) and the cell pellet resuspended in 500μL of PI staining solution (38mM NaCitrate-NaOH pH 7.5, 69μM PI) supplemented with 2μL of 10μg/μL RNase A per tube. Samples were then incubated for 30min at 37°C in the dark before the cells were analyzed with a FACS calibur.

4.31 In vitro Translation and pulldown of in vitro translates with GST fusion proteins

50-70% confluent Sf9 cells were infected with Baculovirus to produce the respective GST fusion protein. After 2-4d, cells were harvested and lysed in 1mL of TNN lyses buffer (50mM Tris-HCl pH 7.5. 250mM NaCl, 5mM EDTA, 0.5% NP-40, 50mM NaF, 1mM DTT, 10μg/mL of aprotinin, 1mM PMSF) for 30min on a head over tail rotator at 4°C. Meanwhile, GSH sepharose beads were precoated with 0.1% nonfat dried milk in NETN buffer (20mM Tris-HCl pH 7.5, 0.5% Nonidet P40, 1mM EDTA, 1M NaCl, 1mM PMSF, 1mM DTT, 10μg/mL of aprotinin) for 10min at 4°C on a head-over-tail rotator and washed three times with NETN buffer. Lysates were centrifuged for 15min at 13.000rpm at 4°C on a table top microcentrifuge and 50μL of 50/50 GSH slurry added to the supernatant. Lysates and beads were incubated at 4°C for 2h on a head-over-tail rotator, centrifuged for 3min at 2000rpm at 4°C on a table top microcentrifuge and washed four times with 1mL TNN buffer before they were finally resuspended in 500μL of TNN buffer. Meanwhile, in vitro-translations with a final volume of 25μL were performed. For that 12.5μL of RRL, 1μL of TNT reaction buffer, 0.5μL of amino acid mixture minus methionine, 0.5μL of RNASIN (40u/μL Promega), 1.5μg of plasmid encoding the to be in vitro expressed protein under the control of a T7 promoter, 0.5μL of TNT T7 RNA polymerase and 2μL of ^{35}S Methionine (1Ci/mmol) were combined with H$_2$O to 25μL and incubated for 1-2h at 37°C. 3μL of IVT samples were then added to the immobilized GST fusion protein and incubated for 1h on a shaker at 4°C. The beads were washed four times with TNN buffer (centrifugation conditions as before) before 30μL of Laemmli's sample buffer was added to elute the proteins from the beads. The samples were boiled for 5min and loaded and separated on a small SDS gel. The gel was stained with colloidal Coomassie ON and destained with dH$_2$O for 1h the next morning, before the gel was scanned using the Odyssey system to confirm equal loading of GST fusion proteins.

The radioactive signal was increased by shaking the gels in EN³HANCE solution (Perkin Elmer) for 45-60min at RT and subsequent washing in dH_2O for 30min at RT. PAGs were dried at 80° for 2h (BIORAD model 583 gel dryer) and exposed to Fuji RX Films (Fuji) for 1-4 weeks. **Fig. 4.1** gives an overview of the whole IVT process.

Fig. 4.1

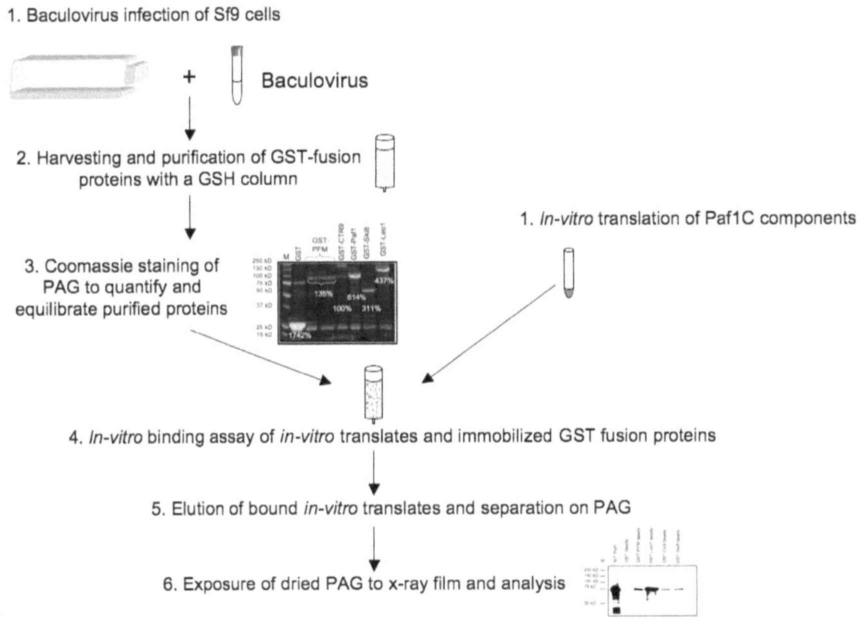

1. Baculovirus infection of Sf9 cells

2. Harvesting and purification of GST-fusion proteins with a GSH column

3. Coomassie staining of PAG to quantify and equilibrate purified proteins

1. In-vitro translation of Paf1C components

4. In-vitro binding assay of in-vitro translates and immobilized GST fusion proteins

5. Elution of bound in-vitro translates and separation on PAG

6. Exposure of dried PAG to x-ray film and analysis

Fig. 4.1: Overview of the IVT process. GST fusion proteins were produced in Baculo-infected *Sf9* cells (step 1) and purified on GSH columns (step 2). To evaluate purifty and determine the quantity of the eluted fusion proteins, eluates were visualized on PAGs by Coomassie staining (step 3). Subsequently, radioactively labeled *in vitro* translated binding candidates were added to the equilibrated amounts of beads and immobilized GST fusion proteins (step 4). After incubation and several washing steps, bound *in vitro* translates were eluted (step 5), concentrated on a PAGE and visualized on an X-ray film.

5 Acknowledgements

Special thanks to all present and past lab members for the nice atmosphere, for the constructive and inspiring discussions, your support and the many positive interactions we have had: Andrea Meyer (for all your insights and also for crossing and keeping the PFM knockout mice), Armelle Yart (for cloning some constructs and your contribution to generate the PFM knockout mouse) Arne, Atilla, Axel, Ayca, Carsten (it is a great experience!), Christiane Wirbelauer (for generating the GST and GST-URI baculovirus), Christian (for our inspiring discussions and exchanges), Christine, Claudia, Claudio, Daniel (it was great fun to have met you here!), Dimitrios, Egon, Grzegorz, Gudrun (for everything:), Ian Frew (thanks also for help with the MEF preparation) Igor (thanks for your great support and our running sessions!), Irina, Ivan, Jean-Philippe (thank you for our running sessions), Jens (crater cake), Julius, Katharina, Katrin B., Katrin E., Madjid, Manuela, Marianne, Melanie, Mojça, Nabil (thanks for the interesting usually late-night exchanges on the state of our planet!), Nan, Peter, Philipp, Pia, Prisca, Prof. Eppenberger, Prof. Jean-Pierre Perriard, Raphael and Charlotte, Renata, Rita und Frau Ferrara (ihr macht einen super job und es war wirklich toll, Euch kennengelernt zu haben!), Rolf, Romeo (thanks for our discussions), Sreya, Susann, Stefan, Stefanie, Strahil, Tatjana and Jaya (also for your help in producing the Adeno-Cre virus), Werner, Yandong, and of course Bogdan Gerya and Felix Hauler for producing and purifying GST-NT-PFM/ GST-CT-PFM in the polyclonal antibody project.

During my studies, I enjoyed and benefited from outstanding teaching performances by a large number of people including Thomas Scheper, Roland Ulber, Bernd Hitzmann, Johannes Refisch, Monika Gedicke, Bernd Walz, Martin Steup, Dieter Fürst, and Anaclet Ngezehayo.

I would like to thank my family and Kristin who supported this thesis on a personal level.

6 Bibliography

Adelman K, Wei W, Ardehali MB, Werner J, Zhu B, Reinberg D & Lis JT 2006 Drosophila Paf1 modulates chromatin structure at actively transcribed genes. *Mol Cell Biol* **26** 250-260.

Akanuma T, Koshida S, Kawamura A, Kishimoto Y & Takada S 2007 Paf1 complex homologues are required for Notch-regulated transcription during somite segmentation. *EMBO Rep* **8** 858-863.

Arnold A, Kim HG, Gaz RD, Eddy RL, Fukushima Y, Byers MG, Shows TB & Kronenberg HM 1989 Molecular cloning and chromosomal mapping of DNA rearranged with the parathyroid hormone gene in a parathyroid adenoma. *J Clin Invest* **83** 2034-2040.

Arranz E, Robledo M, Martinez B, Gallego J, Roman A, Rivas C & Benitez J 1996 Incidence of homogeneously staining regions in non-Hodgkin lymphomas. *Cancer Genet Cytogenet* **87** 1-3.

Bashyam MD, Bair R, Kim YH, Wang P, Hernandez-Boussard T, Karikari CA, Tibshirani R, Maitra A & Pollack JR 2005 Array-based comparative genomic hybridization identifies localized DNA amplifications and homozygous deletions in pancreatic cancer. *Neoplasia* **7** 556-562.

Baxter RC 2000 Insulin-like growth factor (IGF)-binding proteins: interactions with IGFs and intrinsic bioactivities. *Am J Physiol Endocrinol Metab* **278** E967-976.

Bellacosa A, de Feo D, Godwin AK, Bell DW, Cheng JQ, Altomare DA, Wan M, Dubeau L, Scambia G, Masciullo V, et al. 1995 Molecular alterations of the AKT2 oncogene in ovarian and breast carcinomas. *Int J Cancer* **64** 280-285.

Bellacosa A, Kumar CC, Di Cristofano A & Testa JR 2005 Activation of AKT kinases in cancer: implications for therapeutic targeting. *Adv Cancer Res* **94** 29-86.

Bentley DL 2005 Rules of engagement: co-transcriptional recruitment of pre-mRNA processing factors. *Curr Opin Cell Biol* **17** 251-256.

Betz JL, Chang M, Washburn TM, Porter SE, Mueller CL & Jaehning JA 2002 Phenotypic analysis of Paf1/RNA polymerase II complex mutations reveals connections to cell cycle regulation, protein synthesis, and lipid and nucleic acid metabolism. *Mol Genet Genomics* **268** 272-285.

Birkenkamp-Demtroder K, Christensen LL, Olesen SH, Frederiksen CM, Laiho P, Aaltonen LA, Laurberg S, Sorensen FB, Hagemann R & TF OR 2002 Gene expression in colorectal cancer. *Cancer Res* **62** 4352-4363.

Borggrefe T, Davis R, Bareket-Samish A & Kornberg RD 2001 Quantitation of the RNA polymerase II transcription machinery in yeast. *J Biol Chem* **276** 47150-47153.

Bradley KJ, Bowl MR, Williams SE, Ahmad BN, Partridge CJ, Patmanidi AL, Kennedy AM, Loh NY & Thakker RV 2007 Parafibromin is a nuclear protein with a functional monopartite nuclear localization signal. *Oncogene* **26** 1213-1221.

Bradley KJ, Hobbs MR, Buley ID, Carpten JD, Cavaco BM, Fares JE, Laidler P, Manek S, Robbins CM, Salti IS, et al. 2005 Uterine tumours are a phenotypic manifestation of the hyperparathyroidism-jaw tumour syndrome. *Journal Of Internal Medicine* **257** 18-26.

Burgering BM & Kops GJ 2002 Cell cycle and death control: long live Forkheads. *Trends Biochem Sci* **27** 352-360.

Camps J, Armengol G, del Rey J, Lozano JJ, Vauhkonen H, Prat E, Egozcue J, Sumoy L, Knuutila S & Miro R 2006 Genome-wide differences between microsatellite stable and unstable colorectal tumors. *Carcinogenesis* **27** 419-428.

Carling T & Udelsman R 2005 Parathyroid surgery in familial hyperparathyroid disorders*. *J Intern Med* **257** 27-37.

Carpten JD, Robbins CM, Villablanca A, Forsberg L, Presciuttini S, Bailey-Wilson J, Simonds WF, Gillanders EM, Kennedy AM, Chen JD, et al. 2002 HRPT2, encoding parafibromin, is mutated in hyperparathyroidism-jaw tumor syndrome. *Nature Genetics* **32** 676-680.

Carrozza MJ, Li B, Florens L, Suganuma T, Swanson SK, Lee KK, Shia WJ, Anderson S, Yates J, Washburn MP, et al. 2005 Histone H3 methylation by Set2 directs deacetylation of coding regions by Rpd3S to suppress spurious intragenic transcription. *Cell* **123** 581-592.

Cavaco BM, Barros L, Pannett AA, Ruas L, Carvalheiro M, Ruas MM, Krausz T, Santos MA, Sobrinho LG, Leite V, et al. 2001 The hyperparathyroidism-jaw tumour syndrome in a Portuguese kindred. *Qjm* **94** 213-222.

Cavaco BM, Guerra L, Bradley KJ, Carvalho D, Harding B, Oliveira A, Santos MA, Sobrinho LG, Thakker RV & Leite V 2004 Hyperparathyroidism-jaw tumor syndrome in Roma families from Portugal is due to a founder mutation of the HRPT2 gene. *Journal Of Clinical Endocrinology And Metabolism* **89** 1747-1752.

Cavenee WK, Dryja TP, Phillips RA, Benedict WF, Godbout R, Gallie BL, Murphree AL, Strong LC & White RL 1983 Expression of recessive alleles by chromosomal mechanisms in retinoblastoma. *Nature* **305** 779-784.

Cetani F, Pardi E, Borsari S, Viacava P, Dipollina G, Cianferotti L, Ambrogini E, Gazzerro E, Colussi G, Berti P, et al. 2004 Genetic analyses of the HRPT2 gene in primary hyperparathyroidism: germline and somatic mutations in familial and sporadic parathyroid tumors. *J Clin Endocrinol Metab* **89** 5583-5591.

Chang M, French-Cornay D, Fan HY, Klein H, Denis CL & Jaehning JA 1999 A complex containing RNA polymerase II, Paf1p, Cdc73p, Hpr1p, and Ccr4p plays a role in protein kinase C signaling. *Mol Cell Biol* **19** 1056-1067.

Chang MC, Chang YT, Tien YW, Sun CT, Wu MS & Lin JT 2005 Distinct chromosomal aberrations of ampulla of Vater and pancreatic head cancers detected by laser capture microdissection and comparative genomic hybridization. *Oncol Rep* **14** 867-872.

Chaudhary K, Deb S, Moniaux N, Ponnusamy MP & Batra SK 2007 Human RNA polymerase II-associated factor complex: dysregulation in cancer. *Oncogene* **26** 7499-7507.

Cheng JQ, Godwin AK, Bellacosa A, Taguchi T, Franke TF, Hamilton TC, Tsichlis PN & Testa JR 1992 AKT2, a putative oncogene encoding a member of a subfamily of protein-serine/threonine kinases, is amplified in human ovarian carcinomas. *Proc Natl Acad Sci U S A* **89** 9267-9271.

Cheng JQ, Ruggeri B, Klein WM, Sonoda G, Altomare DA, Watson DK & Testa JR 1996 Amplification of AKT2 in human pancreatic cells and inhibition of AKT2 expression and tumorigenicity by antisense RNA. *Proc Natl Acad Sci U S A* **93** 3636-3641.

Cho EJ, Kobor MS, Kim M, Greenblatt J & Buratowski S 2001 Opposing effects of Ctk1 kinase and Fcp1 phosphatase at Ser 2 of the RNA polymerase II C-terminal domain. *Genes Dev* **15** 3319-3329.

Cortajarena AL & Regan L 2006 Ligand binding by TPR domains. *Protein Sci* **15** 1193-1198.

Cryns VL, Rubio MP, Thor AD, Louis DN & Arnold A 1994a p53 abnormalities in human parathyroid carcinoma. *J Clin Endocrinol Metab* **78** 1320-1324.

Cryns VL, Thor A, Xu HJ, Hu SX, Wierman ME, Vickery AL, Jr., Benedict WF & Arnold A 1994b Loss of the retinoblastoma tumor-suppressor gene in parathyroid carcinoma. *N Engl J Med* **330** 757-761.

Curtis LJ, Li Y, Gerbault-Seureau M, Kuick R, Dutrillaux AM, Goubin G, Fawcett J, Cram S, Dutrillaux B, Hanash S, et al. 1998 Amplification of DNA sequences from chromosome 19q13.1 in human pancreatic cell lines. *Genomics* **53** 42-55.

D'Andrea LD & Regan L 2003 TPR proteins: the versatile helix. *Trends Biochem Sci* **28** 655-662.

Djouder N, Metzler SC, Schmidt A, Wirbelauer C, Gstaiger M, Aebersold R, Hess D & Krek W 2007 S6K1-mediated disassembly of mitochondrial URI/PP1gamma complexes activates a negative feedback program that counters S6K1 survival signaling. *Mol Cell* **28** 28-40.

Dorjsuren D, Lin Y, Wei W, Yamashita T, Nomura T, Hayashi N & Murakami S 1998 RMP, a novel RNA polymerase II subunit 5-interacting protein, counteracts transactivation by hepatitis B virus X protein. *Mol Cell Biol* **18** 7546-7555.

Egloff S & Murphy S 2008 Cracking the RNA polymerase II CTD code. *Trends Genet* **24** 280-288.

Firth SM & Baxter RC 2002 Cellular actions of the insulin-like growth factor binding proteins. *Endocr Rev* **23** 824-854.

Ford D, Easton DF, Stratton M, Narod S, Goldgar D, Devilee P, Bishop DT, Weber B, Lenoir G, Chang-Claude J, et al. 1998 Genetic heterogeneity and penetrance analysis of the BRCA1 and BRCA2 genes in breast cancer families. The Breast Cancer Linkage Consortium. *Am J Hum Genet* **62** 676-689.

Foreman PK & Davis RW 1996 CDP1, a novel Saccharomyces cerevisiae gene required for proper nuclear division and chromosome segregation. *Genetics* **144** 1387-1397.

Gerber M & Shilatifard A 2003 Transcriptional elongation by RNA polymerase II and histone methylation. *J Biol Chem* **278** 26303-26306.

Gomes NP, Bjerke G, Llorente B, Szostek SA, Emerson BM & Espinosa JM 2006 Gene-specific requirement for P-TEFb activity and RNA polymerase II phosphorylation within the p53 transcriptional program. *Genes Dev* **20** 601-612.

Gstaiger M, Luke B, Hess D, Oakeley EJ, Wirbelauer C, Blondel M, Vigneron M, Peter M & Krek W 2003 Control of nutrient-sensitive transcription programs by the unconventional prefoldin URI. *Science* **302** 1208-1212.

Hahn MA & Marsh DJ 2005 Identification of a functional bipartite nuclear localization signal in the tumor suppressor parafibromin. *Oncogene* **24** 6241-6248.

Hampsey M & Reinberg D 2003 Tails of intrigue: phosphorylation of RNA polymerase II mediates histone methylation. *Cell* **113** 429-432.

Haven CJ, van Puijenbroek M, Tan MH, Teh BT, Fleuren GJ, van Wezel T & Morreau H 2007 Identification of MEN1 and HRPT2 somatic mutations in paraffin-embedded (sporadic) parathyroid carcinomas. *Clin Endocrinol (Oxf)* **67** 370-376.

Haven CJ, Wong FK, van Dam EW, van der Juijt R, van Asperen C, Jansen J, Rosenberg C, de Wit M, Roijers J, Hoppener J, et al. 2000 A genotypic and histopathological study of a large Dutch kindred with hyperparathyroidism-jaw tumor syndrome. *J Clin Endocrinol Metab* **85** 1449-1454.

He Y, Doyle MR & Amasino RM 2004 PAF1-complex-mediated histone methylation of FLOWERING LOCUS C chromatin is required for the vernalization-responsive, winter-annual habit in Arabidopsis. *Genes Dev* **18** 2774-2784.

Hirano T, Kinoshita N, Morikawa K & Yanagida M 1990 Snap helix with knob and hole: essential repeats in S. pombe nuclear protein nuc2+. *Cell* **60** 319-328.

Howell VM, Haven CJ, Kahnoski K, Khoo SK, Petillo D, Chen J, Fleuren GJ, Robinson BG, Delbridge LW, Philips J, et al. 2003 HRPT2 mutations are associated with malignancy in sporadic parathyroid tumours. *J Med Genet* **40** 657-663.

Hundahl SA, Fleming ID, Fremgen AM & Menck HR 1999 Two hundred eighty-six cases of parathyroid carcinoma treated in the U.S. between 1985-1995: a National Cancer Data Base Report. The American College of Surgeons Commission on Cancer and the American Cancer Society. *Cancer* **86** 538-544.

Imanishi Y, Hosokawa Y, Yoshimoto K, Schipani E, Mallya S, Papanikolaou A, Kifor O, Tokura T, Sablosky M, Ledgard F, et al. 2001 Primary hyperparathyroidism caused by parathyroid-targeted overexpression of cyclin D1 in transgenic mice. *J Clin Invest* **107** 1093-1102.

Iwata T, Mizusawa N, Taketani Y, Itakura M & Yoshimoto K 2007 Parafibromin tumor suppressor enhances cell growth in the cells expressing SV40 large T antigen. *Oncogene* **26** 6176-6183.

Jackson CE, Norum RA, Boyd SB, Talpos GB, Wilson SD, Taggart RT & Mallette LE 1990 Hereditary hyperparathyroidism and multiple ossifying jaw fibromas: a clinically and genetically distinct syndrome. *Surgery* **108** 1006-1012; discussion 1012-1003.

Jensen TH, Dower K, Libri D & Rosbash M 2003 Early formation of mRNP: license for export or quality control? *Mol Cell* **11** 1129-1138.

Jolivet S, Vezon D, Froger N & Mercier R 2006 Non conservation of the meiotic function of the Ski8/Rec103 homolog in Arabidopsis. *Genes Cells* **11** 615-622.

Joshi AA & Struhl K 2005 Eaf3 chromodomain interaction with methylated H3-K36 links histone deacetylation to Pol II elongation. *Mol Cell* **20** 971-978.

Kakinuma A, Morimoto I, Nakano Y, Fujimoto R, Ishida O, Okada Y, Inokuchi N, Fujihira T & Eto S 1994 Familial primary hyperparathyroidism complicated with Wilms' tumor. *Intern Med* **33** 123-126.

Keogh MC, Kurdistani SK, Morris SA, Ahn SH, Podolny V, Collins SR, Schuldiner M, Chin K, Punna T, Thompson NJ, et al. 2005 Cotranscriptional set2 methylation of histone H3 lysine 36 recruits a repressive Rpd3 complex. *Cell* **123** 593-605.

Kerkmann K & Lehming N 2001 Genome-wide expression analysis of a Saccharomyces cerevisiae strain deleted for the Tup1p-interacting protein Cdc73p. *Curr Genet* **39** 284-290.

Knudson AG, Jr. 1971 Mutation and cancer: statistical study of retinoblastoma. *Proc Natl Acad Sci U S A* **68** 820-823.

Koch C, Wollmann P, Dahl M & Lottspeich F 1999 A role for Ctr9p and Paf1p in the regulation G1 cyclin expression in yeast. *Nucleic Acids Res* **27** 2126-2134.

Komarnitsky P, Cho EJ & Buratowski S 2000 Different phosphorylated forms of RNA polymerase II and associated mRNA processing factors during transcription. *Genes Dev* **14** 2452-2460.

Kooijman R 2006 Regulation of apoptosis by insulin-like growth factor (IGF)-I. *Cytokine Growth Factor Rev* **17** 305-323.

Korshunov A, Sycheva R, Gorelyshev S & Golanov A 2005 Clinical utility of fluorescence in situ hybridization (FISH) in nonbrainstem glioblastomas of childhood. *Mod Pathol* **18** 1258-1263.

Krogan NJ, Dover J, Khorrami S, Greenblatt JF, Schneider J, Johnston M & Shilatifard A 2002b COMPASS, a histone H3 (Lysine 4) methyltransferase required for telomeric silencing of gene expression. *J Biol Chem* **277** 10753-10755.

Krogan NJ, Dover J, Wood A, Schneider J, Heidt J, Boateng MA, Dean K, Ryan OW, Golshani A, Johnston M, et al. 2003a The Paf1 complex is required for histone H3 methylation by COMPASS and Dot1p: linking transcriptional elongation to histone methylation. *Mol Cell* **11** 721-729.

Krogan NJ, Kim M, Ahn SH, Zhong G, Kobor MS, Cagney G, Emili A, Shilatifard A, Buratowski S & Greenblatt JF 2002a RNA polymerase II elongation factors of Saccharomyces cerevisiae: a targeted proteomics approach. *Mol Cell Biol* **22** 6979-6992.

Krogan NJ, Kim M, Tong A, Golshani A, Cagney G, Canadien V, Richards DP, Beattie BK, Emili A, Boone C, et al. 2003b Methylation of histone H3 by Set2 in Saccharomyces cerevisiae is linked to transcriptional elongation by RNA polymerase II. *Mol Cell Biol* **23** 4207-4218.

Lamb JR, Tugendreich S & Hieter P 1995 Tetratrico peptide repeat interactions: to TPR or not to TPR? *Trends Biochem Sci* **20** 257-259.

Laribee RN, Krogan NJ, Xiao T, Shibata Y, Hughes TR, Greenblatt JF & Strahl BD 2005 BUR kinase selectively regulates H3 K4 trimethylation and H2B ubiquitylation through recruitment of the PAF elongation complex. *Curr Biol* **15** 1487-1493.

Licatalosi DD, Geiger G, Minet M, Schroeder S, Cilli K, McNeil JB & Bentley DL 2002 Functional interaction of yeast pre-mRNA 3' end processing factors with RNA polymerase II. *Mol Cell* **9** 1101-1111.

Lin L, Czapiga M, Nini L, Zhang JH & Simonds WF 2007 Nuclear localization of the parafibromin tumor suppressor protein implicated in the hyperparathyroidism-jaw tumor syndrome enhances its proapoptotic function. *Mol Cancer Res* **5** 183-193.

Lin L, Zhang JH, Panicker LM & Simonds WF 2008 The parafibromin tumor suppressor protein inhibits cell proliferation by repression of the c-myc proto-oncogene. *Proc Natl Acad Sci U S A* **105** 17420-17425.

Madrona AY & Wilson DK 2004 The structure of Ski8p, a protein regulating mRNA degradation: Implications for WD protein structure. *Protein Sci* **13** 1557-1565.

Mao X, Lillington D, Child F, Russell-Jones R, Young B & Whittaker S 2002 Comparative genomic hybridization analysis of primary cutaneous B-cell lymphomas: identification of common genomic alterations in disease pathogenesis. *Genes Chromosomes Cancer* **35** 144-155.

Marx SJ 2000 Hyperparathyroid and hypoparathyroid disorders. *N Engl J Med* **343** 1863-1875.

Marx SJ, Simonds WF, Agarwal SK, Burns AL, Weinstein LS, Cochran C, Skarulis MC, Spiegel AM, Libutti SK, Alexander HR, Jr., et al. 2002 Hyperparathyroidism in hereditary syndromes: special expressions and special managements. *J Bone Miner Res* **17 Suppl 2** N37-43.

Meinhart A & Cramer P 2004 Recognition of RNA polymerase II carboxy-terminal domain by 3'-RNA-processing factors. *Nature* **430** 223-226.

Miwa W, Yasuda J, Murakami Y, Yashima K, Sugano K, Sekine T, Kono A, Egawa S, Yamaguchi K, Hayashizaki Y, et al. 1996 Isolation of DNA sequences amplified at chromosome 19q13.1-q13.2 including the AKT2 locus in human pancreatic cancer. *Biochem Biophys Res Commun* **225** 968-974.

Mohan S & Baylink DJ 2002 IGF-binding proteins are multifunctional and act via IGF-dependent and -independent mechanisms. *J Endocrinol* **175** 19-31.

Moniaux N, Nemos C, Schmied BM, Chauhan SC, Deb S, Morikane K, Choudhury A, Vanlith M, Sutherlin M, Sikela JM, et al. 2006 The human homologue of the RNA polymerase II-associated factor 1 (hPaf1), localized on the 19q13 amplicon, is associated with tumorigenesis. *Oncogene* **25** 3247-3257.

Mosimann C, Hausmann G & Basler K 2006 Parafibromin/Hyrax activates Wnt/Wg target gene transcription by direct association with beta-catenin/Armadillo. *Cell* **125** 327-341.

Mueller CL & Jaehning JA 2002 Ctr9, Rtf1, and Leo1 are components of the Paf1/RNA polymerase II complex. *Mol Cell Biol* **22** 1971-1980.

Mueller CL, Porter SE, Hoffman MG & Jaehning JA 2004 The Paf1 complex has functions independent of actively transcribing RNA polymerase II. *Mol Cell* **14** 447-456.

Nathrath MH, Kuosaite V, Rosemann M, Kremer M, Poremba C, Wakana S, Yanagi M, Nathrath WB, Hofler H, Imai K, et al. 2002 Two novel tumor suppressor gene loci on chromosome 6q and 15q in human osteosarcoma identified through comparative study of allelic imbalances in mouse and man. *Oncogene* **21** 5975-5980.

Ng HH, Dole S & Struhl K 2003a The Rtf1 component of the Paf1 transcriptional elongation complex is required for ubiquitination of histone H2B. *J Biol Chem* **278** 33625-33628.

Ng HH, Robert F, Young RA & Struhl K 2003b Targeted recruitment of Set1 histone methylase by elongating Pol II provides a localized mark and memory of recent transcriptional activity. *Mol Cell* **11** 709-719.

Ning Y, Schuller AG, Conover CA & Pintar JE 2008 Insulin-like growth factor (IGF) binding protein-4 is both a positive and negative regulator of IGF activity in vivo. *Mol Endocrinol* **22** 1213-1225.

Nordick K, Hoffman MG, Betz JL & Jaehning JA 2008 Direct interactions between the Paf1 complex and a cleavage and polyadenylation factor are revealed by dissociation of Paf1 from RNA polymerase II. *Eukaryot Cell* **7** 1158-1167.

Nordling CO 1953 A new theory on cancer-inducing mechanism. *Br J Cancer* **7** 68-72.

Oh S, Zhang H, Ludwig P & van Nocker S 2004 A mechanism related to the yeast transcriptional regulator Paf1c is required for expression of the Arabidopsis FLC/MAF MADS box gene family. *Plant Cell* **16** 2940-2953.

Parada LA, Hallen M, Tranberg KG, Hagerstrand I, Bondeson L, Mitelman F & Johansson B 1998 Frequent rearrangements of chromosomes 1, 7, and 8 in primary liver cancer. *Genes Chromosomes Cancer* **23** 26-35.

Penheiter KL, Washburn TM, Porter SE, Hoffman MG & Jaehning JA 2005 A posttranscriptional role for the yeast Paf1-RNA polymerase II complex is revealed by identification of primary targets. *Mol Cell* **20** 213-223.

Peterlin BM & Price DH 2006 Controlling the elongation phase of transcription with P-TEFb. *Mol Cell* **23** 297-305.

Pimenta FJ, Gontijo Silveira LF, Tavares GC, Silva AC, Perdigao PF, Castro WH, Gomez MV, Teh BT, De Marco L & Gomez RS 2006 HRPT2 gene alterations in ossifying fibroma of the jaws. *Oral Oncol* **42** 735-739.

Pokholok DK, Hannett NM & Young RA 2002 Exchange of RNA polymerase II initiation and elongation factors during gene expression in vivo. *Mol Cell* **9** 799-809.

Porter SE, Washburn TM, Chang M & Jaehning JA 2002 The yeast paf1-rNA polymerase II complex is required for full expression of a subset of cell cycle-regulated genes. *Eukaryot Cell* **1** 830-842.

Porzionato A, Macchi V, Barzon L, Masi G, Iacobone M, Parenti A, Palu G & De Caro R 2006 Immunohistochemical assessment of parafibromin in mouse and human tissues. *J Anat* **209** 817-827.

Proudfoot N 2004 New perspectives on connecting messenger RNA 3' end formation to transcription. *Curr Opin Cell Biol* **16** 272-278.

Rajaram S, Baylink DJ & Mohan S 1997 Insulin-like growth factor-binding proteins in serum and other biological fluids: regulation and functions. *Endocr Rev* **18** 801-831.

Redeker E, Alders M, Hoovers JM, Richard CW, 3rd, Westerveld A & Mannens M 1995 Physical mapping of 3 candidate tumor suppressor genes relative to Beckwith-Wiedemann syndrome associated chromosomal breakpoints at 11p15.3. *Cytogenet Cell Genet* **68** 222-225.

Rondon AG, Gallardo M, Garcia-Rubio M & Aguilera A 2004 Molecular evidence indicating that the yeast PAF complex is required for transcription elongation. *EMBO Rep* **5** 47-53.

Rozenblatt-Rosen O, Hughes CM, Nannepaga SJ, Shanmugam KS, Copeland TD, Guszczynski T, Resau JH & Meyerson M 2005 The parafibromin tumor suppressor protein is part of a human Paf1 complex. *Molecular And Cellular Biology* **25** 612-620.

Ruggeri BA, Huang L, Wood M, Cheng JQ & Testa JR 1998 Amplification and overexpression of the AKT2 oncogene in a subset of human pancreatic ductal adenocarcinomas. *Mol Carcinog* **21** 81-86.

Schroeder SC, Schwer B, Shuman S & Bentley D 2000 Dynamic association of capping enzymes with transcribing RNA polymerase II. *Genes Dev* **14** 2435-2440.

Schwahn AB 2007 Analyse der Protein-Protein Interaktionen innerhalb des Hefe

PAF1-Komplexes und Untersuchung der Wechselwirkung des

Elongationsfaktors mit yFACT, Casein-Kinase II und Bdf1

als Mittel zur funktionellen Charakterisierung. *Dissertation.*

Selvarajan S, Sii LH, Lee A, Yip G, Bay BH, Tan MH, Teh BT & Tan PH 2008 Parafibromin expression in breast cancer: a novel marker for prognostication? *J Clin Pathol* **61** 64-67.

Shane E 2001 Clinical review 122: Parathyroid carcinoma. *J Clin Endocrinol Metab* **86** 485-493.

Shattuck TM, Valimaki S, Obara T, Gaz RD, Clark OH, Shoback D, Wierman ME, Tojo K, Robbins CM, Carpten JD, et al. 2003 Somatic and germ-line mutations of the HRPT2 gene in sporadic parathyroid carcinoma. *New England Journal Of Medicine* **349** 1722-1729.

Sheldon KE, Mauger DM & Arndt KM 2005 A Requirement for the Saccharomyces cerevisiae Paf1 complex in snoRNA 3' end formation. *Mol Cell* **20** 225-236.

Shi X, Chang M, Wolf AJ, Chang CH, Frazer-Abel AA, Wade PA, Burton ZF & Jaehning JA 1997 Cdc73p and Paf1p are found in a novel RNA polymerase II-containing complex distinct from the Srbp-containing holoenzyme. *Mol Cell Biol* **17** 1160-1169.

Shi X, Finkelstein A, Wolf AJ, Wade PA, Burton ZF & Jaehning JA 1996 Paf1p, an RNA polymerase II-associated factor in Saccharomyces cerevisiae, may have both positive and negative roles in transcription. *Mol Cell Biol* **16** 669-676.

Simonds WF, Robbins CM, Agarwal SK, Hendy GN, Carpten JD & Marx SJ 2004 Familial isolated hyperparathyroidism is rarely caused by germline mutation in HRPT2, the gene for the hyperparathyroidism-jaw tumor syndrome. *Journal Of Clinical Endocrinology And Metabolism* **89** 96-102.

Sitar T, Popowicz GM, Siwanowicz I, Huber R & Holak TA 2006 Structural basis for the inhibition of insulin-like growth factors by insulin-like growth factor-binding proteins. *Proc Natl Acad Sci U S A* **103** 13028-13033.

Sood R, Bonner TI, Makalowska I, Stephan DA, Robbins CM, Connors TD, Morgenbesser SD, Su K, Faruque MU, Pinkett H, et al. 2001 Cloning and characterization of 13 novel transcripts and the human RGS8 gene from the 1q25 region encompassing the hereditary prostate cancer (HPC1) locus. *Genomics* **73** 211-222.

Squazzo SL, Costa PJ, Lindstrom DL, Kumer KE, Simic R, Jennings JL, Link AJ, Arndt KM & Hartzog GA 2002 The Paf1 complex physically and functionally associates with transcription elongation factors in vivo. *Embo J* **21** 1764-1774.

Stange DE, Radlwimmer B, Schubert F, Traub F, Pich A, Toedt G, Mendrzyk F, Lehmann U, Eils R, Kreipe H, et al. 2006 High-resolution genomic profiling reveals association of chromosomal aberrations on 1q and 16p with histologic and genetic subgroups of invasive breast cancer. *Clin Cancer Res* **12** 345-352.

Stolinski LA, Eisenmann DM & Arndt KM 1997 Identification of RTF1, a novel gene important for TATA site selection by TATA box-binding protein in Saccharomyces cerevisiae. *Mol Cell Biol* **17** 4490-4500.

Subramaniam P, Wilkinson S & Shepherd JJ 1995 Inactivation of retinoblastoma gene in malignant parathyroid growths: a candidate genetic trigger? *Aust N Z J Surg* **65** 714-716.

Tan MH, Morrison C, Wang P, Yang X, Haven CJ, Zhang C, Zhao P, Tretiakova MS, Korpi-Hyovalti E, Burgess JR, et al. 2004 Loss of parafibromin immunoreactivity is a distinguishing feature of parathyroid carcinoma. *Clin Cancer Res* **10** 6629-6637.

Tan MH & Teh BT 2004 Renal neoplasia in the hyperparathyroidism-jaw tumor syndrome. *Current Molecular Medicine* **4** 895-897.

Tarkkanen M, Larramendy ML, Bohling T, Serra M, Hattinger CM, Kivioja A, Elomaa I, Picci P & Knuutila S 2006 Malignant fibrous histiocytoma of bone: analysis of genomic imbalances by comparative genomic hybridisation and C-MYC expression by immunohistochemistry. *Eur J Cancer* **42** 1172-1180.

Teh BT, Farnebo F, Kristoffersson U, Sundelin B, Cardinal J, Axelson R, Yap A, Epstein M, Heath H, 3rd, Cameron D, et al. 1996 Autosomal dominant primary hyperparathyroidism and jaw tumor syndrome associated with renal hamartomas and cystic kidney disease: linkage to 1q21-q32 and loss of the wild type allele in renal hamartomas. *J Clin Endocrinol Metab* **81** 4204-4211.

Tenney K, Gerber M, Ilvarsonn A, Schneider J, Gause M, Dorsett D, Eissenberg JC & Shilatifard A 2006 Drosophila Rtf1 functions in histone methylation, gene expression, and Notch signaling. *Proc Natl Acad Sci U S A* **103** 11970-11974.

Velcheti V & Govindan R 2006 Insulin-like growth factor and lung cancer. *J Thorac Oncol* **1** 607-610.

Villablanca A, Calender A, Forsberg L, Hoog A, Cheng JD, Petillo D, Bauters C, Kahnoski K, Ebeling T, Salmela P, et al. 2004 Germline and de novo mutations in the HRPT2 tumour suppressor gene in familial isolated hyperparathyroidism (FIHP). *J Med Genet* **41** e32.

Wade PA, Werel W, Fentzke RC, Thompson NE, Leykam JF, Burgess RR, Jaehning JA & Burton ZF 1996 A novel collection of accessory factors associated with yeast RNA polymerase II. *Protein Expr Purif* **8** 85-90.

Wang P, Bowl MR, Bender S, Peng J, Farber L, Chen J, Ali A, Zhang J, Alberts AS, Thakker RV, et al. 2008 Parafibromin, a component of the human PAF complex, regulates growth factors and is required for embryonic development and survival in adult mice. *Mol Cell Biol*.

Wang PF, Tan MH, Zhang C, Morreau H & Teh BT 2005 HRPT2, a tumor suppressor gene for hyperparathyroidism-jaw tumor syndrome. *Horm Metab Res* **37** 380-383.

Warner J, Epstein M, Sweet A, Singh D, Burgess J, Stranks S, Hill P, Perry-Keene D, Learoyd D, Robinson B, et al. 2004 Genetic testing in familial isolated hyperparathyroidism: unexpected results and their implications. *J Med Genet* **41** 155-160.

Wassif WS, Farnebo F, Teh BT, Moniz CF, Li FY, Harrison JD, Peters TJ, Larsson C & Harris P 1999 Genetic studies of a family with hereditary hyperparathyroidism-jaw tumour syndrome. *Clin Endocrinol (Oxf)* **50** 191-196.

Widner WR & Wickner RB 1993 Evidence that the SKI antiviral system of Saccharomyces cerevisiae acts by blocking expression of viral mRNA. *Mol Cell Biol* **13** 4331-4341.

Wood A, Schneider J, Dover J, Johnston M & Shilatifard A 2003 The Paf1 complex is essential for histone monoubiquitination by the Rad6-Bre1 complex, which signals for histone methylation by COMPASS and Dot1p. *J Biol Chem* **278** 34739-34742.

Woodard GE, Lin L, Zhang JH, Agarwal SK, Marx SJ & Simonds WF 2004 Parafibromin, product of the hyperparathyroidism-jaw tumor syndrome gene HRPT2, regulates cyclin D1/PRAD1 expression. *Oncogene*.

Xiao T, Kao CF, Krogan NJ, Sun ZW, Greenblatt JF, Osley MA & Strahl BD 2005 Histone H2B ubiquitylation is associated with elongating RNA polymerase II. *Mol Cell Biol* **25** 637-651.

Xu X, Sakon M, Nagano H, Hiraoka N, Yamamoto H, Hayashi N, Dono K, Nakamori S, Umeshita K, Ito Y, et al. 2004 Akt2 expression correlates with prognosis of human hepatocellular carcinoma. *Oncol Rep* **11** 25-32.

Yart A, Gstaiger M, Wirbelauer C, Pecnik M, Anastasiou D, Hess D & Krek W 2005 The HRPT2 Tumor Suppressor Gene Product Parafibromin Associates with Human PAF1 and RNA Polymerase II. *Mol Cell Biol* **25** 5052-5060.

Zhang C, Kong D, Tan MH, Pappas DL, Jr., Wang PF, Chen J, Farber L, Zhang N, Koo HM, Weinreich M, et al. 2006 Parafibromin inhibits cancer cell growth and causes G1 phase arrest. *Biochem Biophys Res Commun* **350** 17-24.

Zhao J, Yart A, Frigerio S, Perren A, Schraml P, Weisstanner C, Stallmach T, Krek W & Moch H 2006 Sporadic human renal tumors display frequent allelic imbalances and novel mutations of the HRPT2 gene. *Oncogene*.

Zheng HC, Takahashi H, Li XH, Hara T, Masuda S, Guan YF & Takano Y 2008 Downregulated parafibromin expression is a promising marker for pathogenesis, invasion, metastasis and prognosis of gastric carcinomas. *Virchows Arch* **452** 147-155.

Zhu B, Mandal SS, Pham AD, Zheng Y, Erdjument-Bromage H, Batra SK, Tempst P & Reinberg D 2005a The human PAF complex coordinates transcription with events downstream of RNA synthesis. *Genes Dev* **19** 1668-1673.

Zhu B, Zheng Y, Pham AD, Mandal SS, Erdjument-Bromage H, Tempst P & Reinberg D 2005b Monoubiquitination of human histone H2B: the factors involved and their roles in HOX gene regulation. *Mol Cell* **20** 601-611.

Zhu W, Shiojima I, Ito Y, Li Z, Ikeda H, Yoshida M, Naito AT, Nishi J, Ueno H, Umezawa A, et al. 2008 IGFBP-4 is an inhibitor of canonical Wnt signalling required for cardiogenesis. *Nature* **454** 345-349.

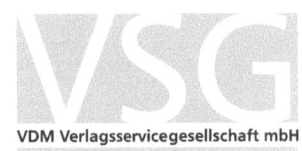

Die VDM Verlagsservicegesellschaft sucht für wissenschaftliche Verlage abgeschlossene und herausragende

Dissertationen, Habilitationen, Diplomarbeiten, Master Theses, Magisterarbeiten usw.

für die kostenlose Publikation als Fachbuch.

Sie verfügen über eine Arbeit, die hohen inhaltlichen und formalen Ansprüchen genügt, und haben Interesse an einer honorarvergüteten Publikation?

Dann senden Sie bitte erste Informationen über sich und Ihre Arbeit per Email an *info@vdm-vsg.de*.

Sie erhalten kurzfristig unser Feedback!

VDM Verlagsservicegesellschaft mbH
Dudweiler Landstr. 99   Telefon +49 681 3720 174
D - 66123 Saarbrücken   Fax   +49 681 3720 1749
www.vdm-vsg.de

Die VDM Verlagsservicegesellschaft mbH vertritt

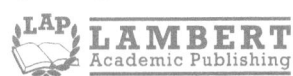
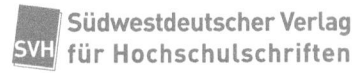

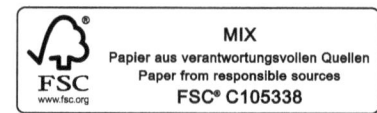

Printed by Books on Demand GmbH, Norderstedt / Germany